Lean & Green

Table of Contents

Introduction

Lean and green diet is a special variant of the low-fat diet, which further makes use of lean proteins instead of fat in promoting weight loss and improving health. Lean protein sources include skinless poultry, fish (e.g. cod and haddock), lean cuts of meat, eggs and vegetable proteins such as lentils and beans. This kind of diet improves the metabolism by increasing the metabolic rate that speeds up weight loss. It also reduces the risk of obesity, because following the lean and green diet does not increase body fat as much as low-fat diets.

The emphasis is on consuming a small amount of meat and fish that are eaten twice a day, together with other protein sources such as eggs, lentils and beans. The diet includes vegetables in addition to fruits that are rich in vitamins (e.g. carrots). The green food includes different varieties of beans like green lentils, black-eyed peas and soybeans. Lean and Green diet is one of the healthy diets that should be consumed frequently, because it complements all other healthy diets.

Recent studies show that lean diets have similar results to low fat diets in reducing body weight. The lean and green diet, however, do not show a considerable improvement in the health risk factors like blood lipids, blood pressure and insulin resistance compared to low-fat diets.

A green lean and cleanse diet, or simply green lean diet, is a diet similar to the concept of a raw food vegan diet, but with less emphasis on raw foods and more emphasis on whole foods that are nonetheless prepared in a way to ensure minimum use of energy during preparation or preservation, for example through the practice of lacto fermentation and cooking at low temperatures under 70 °C (158 °F).

When lean & green food merges with air frying, it can make this diet much easier for people to follow. Air frying food cuts the cooking time in half and makes the food more nutritious.

The Lean and Green diet is a great diet to try. It can help you lose weight and eat healthy foods in the process. The diet practically makes the body burn fats much faster than carbohydrates.

Carbs will be there too, but at far lower levels than before. Foods rich in carbohydrates are the body's primary fuel or the brain's food. (Our bodies turn carbs into glucose.) Because there are hardly any carbohydrates in this diet, the body will have to find a substitute source of energy to keep itself alive.

Once the body realizes that it does not have enough carbohydrates to cover the calories it burns, it turns to fat reserves to provide the required energy. Before that time, the body was using only 15% of its fat reserves for energy—the ratio changes once you start this diet. You will burn fats at a relatively faster rate than fat reserves, and after that, it will burn fat at a relatively faster rate than fat reserves. In this way, the body will find a way to get the required amount of energy from its fat stores keeping the carbs and calories under control.

If you did not change your way of living altogether and added good fats to your diet, it could take carbohydrates. In that case, you might be waiting for at least a year before you will start losing weight with this diet. For you, it is still worth doing this diet. Even if it is yearlong, you will see a great improvement in your overall health. Therefore, when you ingest fats, instead of your body storing them as fat, they are more likely to be converted into a source of energy.

As fat reserves continue to be burned, the body will tend not to gain weight. This is excellent news because fat reserves are not very easy to get rid of completely.

If you ask a nutritionist about this diet, they will recommend it without a doubt. So, if you feel like cleansing your body and starting a diet that will keep you healthy, well-fed, and slender, this diet should be your primary choice.

Engaging into lean and green diet is a good idea to improve not only our health, but also our environment. One should eat less meat products and consume more of fresh fruits and vegetables in order to lower the risk for heart disease and cancer. The latter are mostly linked with meat consumption because of the nitrates located in processed meats. Fruits and vegetables are very low-calorie foods, but they are high in fiber content and rich in vitamins.

The vegetables and fruits that deserve to be consumed are the ones that are grown organically. It is very important to avoid processed foods since they contain a high percentage of fat. Green and lean diet is also linked with the environment preservation. By cutting down meat consumption by at least 50%, we save a lot from greenhouse gas emissions. Considering that meat production requires more energy, it causes more carbon dioxide emissions compared to vegetable production. Another advantage of green and lean diet is improved health care system and lower health problems cost.

Chapter 1. Lean and Green Foods

There are numerous categories of Lean and Green foods that you can eat while following this diet regime.

Green Foods
This section includes all kinds of vegetables that have been categorized from lower, moderate, and high in terms of carbohydrate content. One serving of vegetables should be at ½ cup unless otherwise specified.

Lower Carbohydrate - These are vegetables that contain low amounts of carbohydrates.

- A cup of green leafy vegetables, such as collard greens (raw), lettuce (green leaf, iceberg, butterhead, and romaine), spinach (raw), mustard greens, spring mix, bok choy (raw), and watercress.

- ½ cup of vegetables including cucumbers, celery, radishes, white mushroom, sprouts (mung bean, alfalfa), arugula, turnip greens, escarole, nopales, Swiss chard (raw), jalapeno, and bok choy (cooked).

Moderate Carbohydrate - These are vegetables that contain moderate amounts of carbohydrates.
Below are the types of vegetables that can be consumed in moderation:

- **½ cup of any of the following vegetables** such as asparagus, cauliflower, fennel bulb, eggplant, portabella mushrooms, kale, cooked spinach, summer squash (zucchini and scallop).

Higher Carbohydrates - Foods that are under this category contain a high amount of starch. Make sure to consume limited amounts of these vegetables.

- **½ cup of the following vegetables** like chayote squash, red cabbage, broccoli, cooked collard and mustard greens, green or wax beans, kohlrabi, kabocha squash, cooked leeks, any peppers, okra, raw scallion, summer squash such as straight neck and crookneck, tomatoes, spaghetti squash, turnips, jicama, cooked Swiss chard, and hearts of palm.

Lean Foods

Leanest Foods - These foods are considered to be the leanest as it has only up to 4 grams of total fat. Moreover, dieters should eat a 7-ounce cooked portion of these foods. Consume these foods with 1 healthy fat serving.

- **Fish:** Flounder, cod, haddock, grouper, Mahi, tilapia, tuna (yellowfin fresh or canned), and wild catfish.
- **Shellfish:** Scallops, lobster, crabs, shrimp
- **Game meat:** Elk, deer, buffalo
- **Ground turkey or other meat:** Should be 98% lean **Meatless alternatives:**14 egg whites, 2 cups egg
- substitute, 5 ounces seitan, 1 ½ cups 1% cottage cheese, and 12 ounces non-fat 0% Greek yogurt

Leaner Foods - These foods contain 5 to 9 grams of total fat. Consume these foods with 1 healthy fat serving. Make sure to consume only 6 ounces of a cooked portion of these foods daily:

- **Fish:** Halibut, trout, and swordfish

  Chicken: White meat such as breasts as long as the skin
- is removed
- **Turkey:** Ground turkey as long as it is 95% to 97% lean.

  Meatless options:2 whole eggs plus 4 egg whites, 2
- whole eggs plus one cup egg substitute, 1 ½ cups 2% cottage cheese, and 12 ounces low fat 2% plain Greek yogurt

Lean Foods - These are foods that contain 10g to 20g total fat. When consuming these foods, there should be no serving of healthy fat. These include the following:

  Fish: Tuna (Bluefin steak), salmon, herring, farmed
- catfish, and mackerel
- **Lean beef:** Ground, steak, and roast
- **Lamb:** All cuts

  Pork: Pork chops, pork tenderloin, and all parts. Make
- sure to remove the skin
- **Ground turkey and other meats:**85% to 94% lean
- **Chicken:** Any dark meat

- **Meatless options:** 15 ounces extra-firm tofu, 3 whole eggs (up to two times per week), 4 ounces reduced-fat skim cheese, 8 ounces part-skim ricotta cheese, and 5 ounces tempeh

Healthy Fat Servings - Healthy fat servings are allowed under this diet. They should contain 5 grams of fat and less than grams of carbohydrates. Make sure that you add between 0 and 2 healthy fat servings daily. Below are the different healthy fat servings that you can eat:

- 1 teaspoon oil (any kind of oil)
- 1 tablespoon low carbohydrate salad dressing
- 2 tablespoons reduced-fat salad dressing
- 5 to 10 black or green olives
- 1 ½ ounce avocado
- 1/3-ounce plain nuts including peanuts, almonds, pistachios
- 1 tablespoon plain seeds such as chia, sesame, flax, and pumpkin seeds
- ½ tablespoon regular butter, mayonnaise, and margarine

Lean & Green Recipes

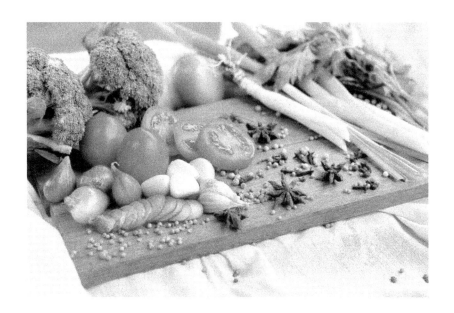

Chapter 2. Breakfast Recipes

1. Sun-Dried Tomato Garlic Bruschetta
Preparation Time: 10 Minutes
Cooking Time: 5 Minutes
Servings: 6
Ingredients:

- 2 Slices sourdough bread, toasted
- 1 Tsp. Chives, minced
- 1 Garlic clove, peeled
- 2 Tsp. Sun-dried tomatoes in olive oil, minced
- 1 Tsp. Olive oil

Directions:

1. Vigorously rub garlic clove on one side of each of the toasted bread slices
2. Spread equal portions of sun-dried tomatoes on the garlic side of the bread. Sprinkle chives and drizzle olive oil on top.
3. Pop both slices into an oven toaster, and cook until well heated through.
4. Place bruschetta on a plate. Serve warm.

Nutrition:

- Calories: 149 kcal
- Protein: 6.12g
- Fat: 2.99g
- Carbohydrates: 24.39g

2. Gingerbread Oatmeal Breakfast

Preparation Time: 10 Minutes
Cooking Time: 0 Minutes
Servings: 4
Ingredients:

- 1 cup steel-cut oats
- 4 cups drinking water
- Organic Maple syrup, to taste
- 1 Tsp. Ground cloves
- 1 ½ Tbsp. Ground cinnamon
- 1/8 Tsp. Nutmeg
- ¼ Tsp. Ground ginger
- ¼ Tsp. Ground coriander
- ¼ Tsp. Ground allspice
- ¼ Tsp. Ground cardamom
- Fresh mixed berries

Directions:

1. Cook the oats based on the package instructions. When it comes to a boil, reduce heat and simmer.
2. Stir in all the spices and continue cooking until cooked to desired doneness.
3. Serve in four serving bowls and drizzle with maple syrup and top with fresh berries.
4. Enjoy!

Nutrition:

- Calories: 87 kcal
- Protein: 5.82g
- Fat: 3.26g
- Carbohydrates: 18.22g

3. Oat Porridge With Cherry & Coconut

Preparation Time: 10 Minutes
Cooking Time: 0 Minutes
Servings: 3
Ingredients:

- 1 ½ Cups regular oats
- 3 cups coconut milk
- 4 Tbsp. Chia seed
- 3 Tbsp. Raw cacao
- Coconut shavings
- Dark chocolate shavings
- Fresh or frozen tart cherries
- A pinch of stevia, optional
- Maple syrup, to taste (optional)

Directions:

1. Combine the oats, milk, stevia, and cacao in a medium saucepan over medium heat and bring to a boil. Lower the heat, then simmer until the oats are cooked to desired doneness.
2. Divide the porridge among three serving bowls and top with dark chocolate, chia seeds, and coconut shavings, cherries, and a little drizzle of maple syrup.

Nutrition:

- Calories: 343 kcal
- Protein: 15.64g
- Fat: 12.78g
- Carbohydrates: 41.63g

4. Hash Browns

Preparation Time: 15 Minutes
Cooking Time: 15 Minutes
Servings: 4
Ingredients:

- 1 pound russet potatoes, peeled, processed using a grater
- Pinch of sea salt
- Pinch of black pepper, to taste
- 3 Tbsp. Olive oil

Directions:

1. Line a microwave safe-dish with paper towels. Spread shredded potatoes on top—microwave veggies on the highest heat setting for 2 minutes. Remove from heat.
2. Pour one tablespoon of oil into a non-stick skillet set over medium heat.
3. Cooking in batches, place a generous pinch of potatoes into the hot oil. Press down using the back of a spatula.
4. Cook for 3 minutes on every side, or until brown and crispy. Drain on paper towels—repeat the step for the remaining potatoes. Add more oil as needed.
5. Season with salt and pepper. Serve.

Nutrition:

- Calories: 200 kcal
- Protein: 4.03g
- Fat: 11.73g
- Carbohydrates: 20.49g

5. Apple Ginger and Rhubarb Muffins

Preparation Time: 15 Minutes
Cooking Time: 25 Minutes
Servings: 4
Ingredients:

- ½ Cup Finely ground almonds
- ¼ Cup Brown rice flour
- ½ Cup Buckwheat flour
- 1/8 Cup Unrefined raw sugar
- 2 Tbsp. Arrowroot flour
- 1 Tbsp. Linseed meal
- 2 Tbsp. Crystallized ginger, finely chopped
- ½ Tsp. Ground ginger
- ½ Tsp. Ground cinnamon
- 2 Tsp. Gluten-free baking powder
- A pinch of fine sea salt
- 1 small apple, peeled and finely diced
- 1 cup finely chopped rhubarb
- 1/3 cup almond/ rice milk
- 1 Large egg
- ¼ cup extra virgin olive oil
- 1 Tsp. Pure vanilla extract

Directions:

1. Set your oven to 350°F grease an eight-cup muffin tin and line with paper cases.
2. Combine the almond four, linseed meal, ginger, salt, and sugar in a mixing bowl. Sieve this mixture over the other flours, spices, and baking powder and use a whisk to combine well.
3. Stir in the apple and rhubarb in the flour mixture until evenly coated.
4. In a separate bowl, whisk the milk, vanilla, and egg, then pour it into the dry mixture. Stir until just combined — don't overwork the batter as this can yield very tough muffins.
5. Grease a muffin pan with oil. Scoop the mixture and top with a few slices of rhubarb. Bake for at least 25 minutes till they start turning golden or when an inserted toothpick emerges clean.
6. Take off from the oven and let sit for at least 5 minutes before transferring the muffins to a wire rack for further cooling.
7. Serve warm with a glass of squeezed juice.
8. Enjoy!

Nutrition:

- Calories: 325 kcal
- Protein: 6.32g
- Fat: 9.82g
- Carbohydrates: 55.71g

6. Anti-Inflammatory Breakfast Frittata

Preparation Time: 10 Minutes
Cooking Time: 40 Minutes
Servings: 4
Ingredients:

- 4 large eggs
- 6 Egg whites
- 450g Button mushrooms
- 450g Baby spinach
- 125g Firm tofu
- 1 Onion, chopped
- 1 Tbsp. Minced garlic
- ½ Tsp. Ground turmeric
- ½ Tsp. Cracked black pepper
- ¼ Cup water
- Kosher salt to taste

Directions:

1. Set your oven to 350°F.
2. Sauté the mushrooms in a little bit of extra virgin olive oil in a large non-stick ovenproof pan over medium heat. Add the onions once the mushrooms start turning golden and cook for 3 minutes until the onions become soft.
3. Stir in the garlic, then cook for at least 30 seconds until fragrant before adding the spinach. Pour in water, cover, and cook until the spinach becomes wilted for about 2 minutes.
4. Take off the lid and continue cooking up until the water evaporates. Now, combine the eggs, egg whites, tofu, pepper, turmeric, and salt in a bowl. When all the liquid has evaporated, pour in the egg mixture, let cook for about 2 minutes until the edges start setting, then transfer to the oven and bake for about 25 minutes or until cooked.

5. Take off from the oven, then let sit for at least 5 minutes before cutting it into quarters and serving.
6. Enjoy!

- **Tip:** Baby spinach and mushrooms boost the nutrient profile of the eggs to provide you with amazing anti-inflammatory benefits.

Nutrition:

- Calories: 521 kcal
- Protein: 29.13g
- Fat: 10.45g
- Carbohydrates: 94.94g

7. White and Green Quiche

Preparation Time: 10 Minutes
Cooking Time: 40 Minutes
Servings: 3
Ingredients:

- 3 Cups of fresh spinach, chopped
- 15 Large free-range eggs
- 3 Cloves of garlic, minced
- 5 White mushrooms, sliced
- 1 Small sized onion, finely chopped
- 1 ½ Teaspoon of baking powder
- Ground black pepper to taste
- 1 ½ Cups of coconut milk
- Ghee, as required to grease the dish
- Sea salt to taste

Directions:

1. Set the oven to 350°F.
2. Get a baking dish, then grease it with organic ghee.
3. Break all the eggs in a huge bowl, then whisk well.
4. Stir in coconut milk. Beat well
5. While you are whisking the eggs, start adding the remaining ingredients to them.
6. When all the ingredients are thoroughly blended, pour all of it into the prepared baking dish.
7. Bake for at least 40 minutes; up to the quiche is set in the middle.
8. Enjoy!

Nutrition:

- Calories: 608 kcal
- Protein: 20.28g
- Fat: 53.42g
- Carbohydrates: 16.88g

8. Yummy Steak Muffins

Preparation Time: 10 Minutes
Cooking Time: 20 Minutes
Servings: 4
Ingredients:

- 1 Cup red bell pepper, diced
- 2 Tablespoons of water
- 8 Ounces thin steak, cooked and finely chopped
- ¼ Teaspoon of sea salt
- Dash of freshly ground black pepper
- 8 Free-range eggs
- 1 Cup of finely diced onion

Directions:

1. Set the oven to 350°F
2. Take eight muffin tins and line them with parchment paper liners.
3. Get a large bowl and crack all the eggs in it.
4. Beat well the eggs.
5. Blend in all the remaining ingredients.
6. Spoon the batter into the arrange muffin tins. Fill three-fourth of each tin.
7. Put the muffin tins in the preheated oven for about 20 minutes, until the muffins are baked and set in the middle.
8. Enjoy!

Nutrition:

- Calories: 151 kcal
- Protein: 17.92g
- Fat: 7.32g
- Carbohydrates: 3.75g

9. Breakfast Sausage and Mushroom Casserole

Preparation Time: 20 Minutes
Cooking Time: 45 Minutes
Servings: 4
Ingredients:

- 450g of Italian sausage, cooked and crumbled
- ¾ Cup of coconut milk
- 8 Ounces of white mushrooms, sliced
- 1 Medium onion, finely diced
- 2 Tablespoons of organic ghee
- 6 Free-range eggs
- 600g of sweet potatoes
- 1 Red bell pepper, roasted
- 3/4 Tsp. of ground black pepper, divided
- 1 ½ Tsp. of sea salt, divided

Directions:

1. Peel and shred the sweet potatoes.
2. Take a bowl, fill it with ice-cold water, and soak the sweet potatoes in it. Set aside.
3. Peel the roasted bell pepper, remove its seeds and finely dice it.
4. Set the oven to 375°F.
5. Get a casserole baking dish and grease it with organic ghee.
6. Put a skillet over medium flame and cook the mushrooms in it. Cook until the mushrooms are crispy and brown.
7. Take the mushrooms out and mix them with the crumbled sausage.
8. Now sauté the onions in the same skillet. Cook up to the onions are soft and golden. This should take about 4–5 minutes.
9. Take the onions out and mix them in the sausage-mushroom mixture.
10. Add the diced bell pepper to the same mixture.
11. Mix well and set aside for a while.
12. Now drain the soaked shredded potatoes, put them on a paper towel, and pat dry.
13. Bring the sweet potatoes to a bowl and add about a teaspoon of salt and half a teaspoon of ground black pepper to it. Mix well and set aside.
14. Now take a large bowl and crack the eggs in it.
15. Break the eggs and then blend in the coconut milk.

16. Stir in the remaining black pepper and salt.
17. Take the greased casserole dish and spread the seasoned sweet potatoes evenly in the base of the dish.
18. Next, spread the sausage mixture evenly in the dish.
19. Finally, spread the egg mixture.
20. Now cover the casserole dish using a piece of aluminum foil.
21. Bake for 20-30 minutes. To check if the casserole is baked properly, insert a tester in the middle of the casserole, and it should come out clean.
22. Uncover the casserole dish and bake it again, uncovered for 5 -10 minutes, until the casserole is a little golden on the top.
23. Allow it to cool for 10 minutes.
24. Enjoy!

Nutrition:

- Calories: 598 kcal
- Protein: 28.65g
- Fat: 36.75g
- Carbohydrates: 48.01g

10. Mushroom Crêpes

Preparation Time: 1 Hour 30 minutes
Cooking Time: 30 Minutes
Servings: 6
Ingredients:

- 2 Eggs
- 3/4 Cup milk
- ½ Cup all-purpose flour
- 1/4 Teaspoon salt

For the filling:

- 3 Tablespoons all-purpose flour
- 2 cups of cremini mushrooms, sliced
- 3/4 cup chicken broth
- ½ Cup Parmesan cheese, grated
- 1/8 Teaspoon cayenne
- 1/8 Teaspoon nutmeg
- ¾ Cup milk
- 3 Garlic cloves, minced
- 2 Tablespoons of parsley (chopped)
- 6 Slices of deli-sliced cooked lean ham
- 1/4 Teaspoon of salt
- Freshly ground pepper

Directions:

1. Put and combine the salt and flour in a bowl. In another bowl, whisk the eggs and milk. Gradually combine the two mixtures until smooth. Leave for 15 minutes.
2. Spray a skillet using non-stick cooking spray and put it over medium heat. Stir the batter a little. Add 1/4 of the batter into the skillet. Tilt the skillet to form a thin and even crêpe. Cook for 1-2 minutes or until the bottom is golden and the top is set. Flip and cook for 20 seconds. Transfer to a plate.
3. Repeat the steps with the remaining batter. Loosely cover the cooked crêpes with plastic wrap.
4. Put all the ingredients together for filling in a saucepan on medium heat — flour, milk, cayenne, nutmeg, and pepper. Constantly whisk until thick or around 7 minutes. Remove from the stove. Stir in a tablespoon of parsley and cheese. Loosely cover to keep warm.
5. Spray a skillet using non-stick cooking spray and put over medium heat. Cook the garlic and mushrooms. Season with

salt. Cook for 6 minutes or until the mushrooms are soft. Add two tablespoons of sherry—Cook for a couple of minutes. Remove from the stove. Add the remaining parsley and stir.

6. Put the crêpes side by side on a flat surface. Spread a tablespoon of the sauce and two tablespoons of the cooked mushrooms. Roll up the crêpes and transfer them to a greased baking dish. Put all the sauce on top—Bake in the oven at 450°F for 15 minutes.

Nutrition:

- Calories: 232 kcal
- Protein: 16.51g
- Fat: 10.8g
- Carbohydrates: 16.25g

11. Beef Breakfast Casserole

Preparation Time: 10 Minutes
Cooking Time: 30 Minutes
Servings: 5
Ingredients:

- 1 Pound of ground beef, cooked
- 10 Eggs
- ½ Cup Pico de Gallo
- 1 Cup baby spinach
- ¼ Cup sliced black olives
- Freshly ground black pepper

Directions:

1. Preheat oven to 350 degrees Fahrenheit. Prepare a 9" glass pie plate with non-stick spray.
2. Whisk the eggs until frothy—season with salt and pepper.
3. Layer the cooked ground beef, Pico de Gallo, and spinach on the pie plate.
4. Slowly pour the eggs over the top.
5. Top with black olives.
6. Bake for at least 30 minutes until firm in the middle.
7. Slice into five pieces and serve.

Nutrition:

- Calories: 479 kcal
- Protein: 43.54g
- Fat: 30.59g
- Carbohydrates: 4.65g

12. Fantastic Spaghetti Squash With Cheese and Basil Pesto

Preparation Time: 10 Minutes
Cooking Time: 35 Minutes
Servings: 2
Ingredients:

- 1 Cup cooked spaghetti squash, drained
- Salt, to taste
- Freshly cracked black pepper, to taste
- ½ Tbsp. olive oil
- ¼ Cup ricotta cheese, unsweetened
- 2 oz. Fresh mozzarella cheese, cubed
- 1/8 Cup basil pesto

Directions:

1. Switch on the oven, then set its temperature to 375°F and let it preheat.
2. Meanwhile, take a medium bowl, add spaghetti squash in it and then season with salt and black pepper.
3. Take a casserole dish, grease it with oil, add squash mixture in it, top it with ricotta cheese and mozzarella cheese and bake for 10 minutes until cooked.
4. When done, remove the casserole dish from the oven, drizzle pesto on top and serve immediately.

Nutrition:

- Calories: 169
- Total Fat: 11.3g
- Total Carbs: 6.2g
- Protein: 11.9g
- Sugar: 0.1g
- Sodium 217mg

13. Ham and Veggie Frittata Muffins

Preparation Time: 10 Minutes
Cooking Time: 25 Minutes
Servings: 12
Ingredients:

- 5 Ounces thinly sliced ham
- 8 Large eggs
- 4 Tablespoons coconut oil
- ½ Yellow onion, finely diced
- 8 oz. Frozen spinach, thawed and drained
- 8 oz. Mushrooms, thinly sliced
- 1 Cup cherry tomatoes, halved
- ¼ Cup coconut milk (canned)
- 2 Tablespoons coconut flour
- Sea salt and pepper to taste

Directions:

1. Preheat oven to 375 degrees Fahrenheit.
2. In a medium skillet, warm the coconut oil on medium heat. Add the onion and cook until softened.
3. Add the mushrooms, spinach, and cherry tomatoes. Season with salt and pepper. Cook until the mushrooms have softened. About 5 minutes. Remove from heat and set aside.
4. In a huge bowl, beat the eggs together with coconut milk and coconut flour. Stir in the cooled veggie mixture.
5. Line each cavity of a 12 cavity muffin tin with the thinly sliced ham. Pour the egg mixture into each one and bake for 20 minutes.
6. Remove from oven and allow to cool for about 5 minutes before transferring to a wire rack.

- **Tip:** It's important to maximize the benefit of a vegetable-rich diet to eat a variety of colors, and these veggie-packed frittata muffins do just that. The onion, spinach, mushrooms, and cherry tomatoes provide a wide range of vitamins and nutrients and a healthy dose of fiber.

Nutrition:

- Calories: 125 kcal
- Protein: 5.96g
- Fat: 9.84g
- Carbohydrates: 4.48g

14. Cheesy Flax and Hemp Seeds Muffins

Preparation Time: 5 Minutes
Cooking Time: 30 Minutes
Servings: 2
Ingredients:

- 1/8 Cup flax seeds meal
- ¼ Cup raw hemp seeds
- ¼ Cup almond meal
- Salt, to taste
- ¼ Tsp. Baking powder
- 3 Organic eggs, beaten
- 1/8 Cup nutritional yeast flakes
- ¼ Cup cottage cheese, low-fat
- ¼ Cup grated parmesan cheese
- ¼ Cup scallion, sliced thinly
- 1 Tbsp. Olive oil

Directions:

1. Switch on the oven, then set it to 360°F and let it preheat.
2. Meanwhile, take two ramekins, grease them with oil, and set them aside until required.
3. Take a medium bowl, add flax seeds, hemp seeds, and almond meal, and then stir in salt and baking powder until mixed.
4. Crack eggs in another bowl, add yeast, cottage cheese, and parmesan, stir well until combined, and then stir this mixture into the almond meal mixture until incorporated.
5. Fold in scallions, then distribute the mixture between prepared ramekins and bake for 30 minutes until muffins are firm and the top is nicely golden brown.
6. When done, take out the muffins from the ramekins and let them cool completely on a wire rack.
7. For meal prepping, wrap each muffin with a paper towel and refrigerate for up to thirty-four days.
8. When ready to eat, reheat muffins in the microwave until hot and then serve.

Nutrition:

- Calories: 179
- Total Fat: 10.9g
- Total Carbs: 6.9g
- Protein: 15.4g
- Sugar: 2.3g
- Sodium: 311mg

15. Cheddar and Chive Souffles

Preparation Time: 10 Minutes
Cooking Time: 25 Minutes
Servings: 8
Ingredients:

- ½ Cup almond flour
- ¼ Cup chopped chives
- 1 Tsp. salt
- ½ Tsp. xanthan gum
- 1 Tsp. ground mustard
- ¼ Tsp. cayenne pepper
- ½ Tsp. cracked black pepper
- ¾ Cup heavy cream
- 2 Cups shredded cheddar cheese
- ½ Cup baking powder
- 6 Organic eggs, separated

Directions:

1. Switch on the oven, then set its temperature to 350°F and let it preheat.
2. Take a medium bowl, add flour in it, add remaining ingredients, except for baking powder and eggs, and whisk until combined.
3. Separate egg yolks and egg whites between two bowls, add egg yolks in the flour mixture, and whisk until incorporated.
4. Add baking powder into the egg whites and beat with an electric mixer until stiff peaks form, and then stir egg whites into the flour mixture until well mixed.
5. Divide the batter evenly between eight ramekins and then bake for 25 minutes until done.
6. Serve straight away or store in the refrigerator until ready to eat.

Nutrition:

- Calories: 288
- Total Fat: 21g
- Total Carbs: 3g
- Protein: 14g

16. Shirataki Pasta With Avocado and Cream

Preparation Time: 10 Minutes
Cooking Time: 6 Minutes
Servings: 2
Ingredients:

- ½ Packet of shirataki noodles, cooked
- ½ Avocado
- ½ Tsp. cracked black pepper
- ½ Tsp. salt
- ½ Tsp. dried basil
- 1/8 Cup heavy cream

Directions:

1. Place a medium pot half full with water over medium heat, bring it to boil, then add noodles and cook for 2 minutes.
2. Then drain the noodles and set them aside until required.
3. Place avocado in a bowl, mash it with a fork,
4. Mash avocado in a bowl, transfer it to a blender, add remaining ingredients, and pulse until smooth.
5. Take a frying pan, place it over medium heat and when hot, add noodles in it, pour in the avocado mixture, stir well and cook for 2 minutes until hot.
6. Serve straight away.

Nutrition:

- Calories: 131
- Total Fat: 12.6g
- Total Carbs: 4.9g
- Protein: 1.2g
- Sugar: 0.3g
- Sodium: 588mg

17. Mango Granola

Preparation Time: 10 Minutes
Cooking Time: 30 Minutes
Servings: 4
Ingredients:

- 2 Cups rolled oats
- 1 Cup dried mango, chopped
- ½ Cup almonds, roughly chopped
- ½ Cup nuts
- ½ Cup dates, roughly chopped
- 3 Tbsp. Sesame seeds
- 2 Tsp. Cinnamon
- 2/3 Cups agave nectar
- 2 Tbsp. Coconut oil
- 2 Tbsp. Water

Directions:

1. Set the oven at 320°F
2. In a large bowl, put the oats, almonds, nuts, sesame seeds, dates, and cinnamon, then mix well.
3. Meanwhile, heat a saucepan over medium heat, pour in the agave syrup, coconut oil, and water.
4. Stir and let it cook for at least 3 minutes or until the coconut oil has melted.
5. Gradually pour the syrup mixture into the bowl with the oats and nuts and stir well, ensure that all the ingredients are coated with the syrup.
6. Transfer the granola to a baking sheet lined with parchment paper and place in the oven to bake for 20 minutes.
7. After 20 minutes, take off the tray from the oven and lay the chopped dried mango on top. Put back in the oven, then bake again for another 5 minutes.
8. Let the granola cool to room temperature before serving or placing it in an airtight container for storage. The shelf life of the granola will last up to 2-3 weeks.

Nutrition:

- Calories: 434 kcal
- Protein: 13.16g
- Fat: 28.3g
- Carbohydrates: 55.19g

18. Blueberry & Cashew Waffles

Preparation Time: 15 Minutes
Cooking Time: 4-5 Minutes
Servings: 5
Ingredients:

- 1 Cup raw cashews
- 3 Tablespoons coconut flour
- 1 Tsp. Baking soda
- Salt, to taste
- ½ Cup unsweetened almond milk
- 3 Organic eggs
- ¼ Cup coconut oil, melted
- 3 Tablespoons organic honey
- ½ Teaspoon organic vanilla flavor
- 1 Cup fresh blueberries

Directions:

1. Preheat the waffle iron, after which grease it.
2. In a mixer, add cashews and pulse till flour-like consistency forms.
3. Transfer the cashew flour to a big bowl.
4. Add almond flour, baking soda, and salt and mix well.
5. In another bowl, put the remaining ingredients and beat till well combined.
6. Put the egg mixture into the flour mixture, then mix till well combined.
7. Fold in blueberries.
8. In the preheated waffle iron, add the required amount of mixture.
9. Cook for around 4-5 minutes.
10. Repeat with the remaining mixture.

Nutrition:

- Calories: 432
- Fat: 32
- Carbohydrates: 32g
- Protein: 13g

19. Tomato and Avocado Omelet

Preparation Time: 5 Minutes
Cooking Time: 5 Minutes
Servings: 1
Ingredients:

- 2 Eggs
- ¼ avocado, diced
- 4 Cherry tomatoes, halved
- 1 tablespoon cilantro, chopped
- Squeezed lime juice
- Pinch of salt

Directions:

1. Put together the avocado, tomatoes, cilantro, lime juice, and salt in a small bowl, then mix well and set aside.
2. Warm a medium non-stick skillet on medium heat, whisk the eggs until frothy and add to the pan. Move the eggs around gently with a rubber spatula until they begin to set.
3. Scatter the avocado mixture over half of the omelet. Remove from heat, and slide the omelet onto a plate as you fold it in half.
4. Serve immediately.

Nutrition:

- Calories: 433 kcal
- Protein: 25.55g
- Fat: 32.75g
- Carbohydrates: 10.06g

20. Vegan-Friendly Banana Bread

Preparation Time: 15 Minutes
Cooking Time: 40 Minutes
Servings: 4-6
Ingredients:

- 2 Ripe bananas, mashed
- 1/3 Cup brewed coffee
- 3 Tbsp. Chia seeds
- 6 Tbsp. Water
- ½ Cup soft vegan butter
- ½ Cup maple syrup
- 2 Cups flour
- 2 Tsp. Baking powder
- 1 Tsp. Cinnamon powder
- 1 Tsp. Allspice
- ½ Tsp. Salt

Directions:

1. Set the oven at 350°F.
2. Bring the chia seeds in a small bowl, then soak them with 6 Tbsp. of water. Stir well and set aside.
3. In a mixing bowl, mix using a hand mixer the vegan butter and maple syrup until it turns fluffy. Add the chia seeds along with the mashed bananas.
4. Mix well, and then add the coffee.
5. Meanwhile, sift all the dry ingredients (flour, baking powder, cinnamon powder, allspice, and salt) and then gradually add into the bowl with the wet ingredients.
6. Combine the ingredients well, and then pour over a baking pan lined with parchment paper.
7. Place in the oven to bake for at least 30-40 minutes or until the toothpick comes out clean after inserting in the bread.
8. Allow the bread to cool before serving.

Nutrition:

- Calories: 371 kcal
- Protein: 5.59g
- Fat: 16.81g
- Carbohydrates: 49.98g

Chapter 3. Side Dish Recipes

21. Plant-Powered Pancakes

Preparation Time: 5 Minutes
Cooking Time: 15 Minutes
Servings: 8
Ingredients:

- 1 Cup whole-wheat flour
- 1 Teaspoon baking powder
- ½ Teaspoon ground cinnamon
- 1 Cup plant-based milk
- ½ Cup unsweetened applesauce
- 1/4 Cup maple syrup
- 1 Teaspoon vanilla extract

Directions:

1. In a large bowl, combine the flour, baking powder, and cinnamon.
2. Stir in the milk, applesauce, maple syrup, and vanilla until no dry flour is left and the batter is smooth.
3. Heat a large, nonstick skillet or griddle over medium heat. For each pancake, pour 1/4 cup of batter onto the hot skillet. Once bubbles form over the top of the pancake and the sides begin to brown, flip and cook for 1 or 2 minutes more.
4. Repeat until the entire batter is used, and serve.

Nutrition:

- Fat: 2g
- Carbohydrates: 44g
- Fiber: 5g
- Protein: 5g

22. Hemp Seed Porridge

Preparation Time: 5 Minutes
Cooking Time: 5 Minutes
Servings: 6
Ingredients:

- 3 Cups cooked hemp seed
- 1 Packet Stevia
- 1 Cup coconut milk

Directions:

1. In a saucepan, mix the seeds and the coconut milk over moderate heat for about 5 minutes as you stir it constantly.
2. Remove the pan from the burner, then add the Stevia. Stir.
3. Serve in 6 bowls.
4. Enjoy.

Nutrition:

- Calories: 236 kcal
- Fat: 1.8g
- Carbs: 48.3g
- Protein: 7g

23. Walnut Crunch Banana Bread

Preparation Time: 5 minutes
Cooking Time: 1 hour and 30 minutes
Servings: 1
Ingredients:

- 4 Ripe bananas
- 1/4 Cup maple syrup
- 1 Tablespoon apple cider vinegar
- 1 Teaspoon vanilla extract
- 1½ Cups whole-wheat flour
- ½ Teaspoon ground cinnamon
- ½ Teaspoon baking soda
- 1/4 Cup walnut pieces (optional)

Directions:

1. Preheat the oven to 350°F.
2. In a large bowl, use a fork or mixing spoon to mash the bananas until they reach a puréed consistency (small bits of banana are acceptable). Stir in the maple syrup, apple cider vinegar, and vanilla.
3. Stir in the flour, cinnamon, and baking soda. Fold in the walnut pieces (if using).
4. Gently pour the batter into a loaf pan, filling it no more than three-quarters of the way full, bake for 1 hour, or until you can stick a knife into the middle and it comes out clean.
5. Remove from the oven and allow cooling on the countertop for a minimum of 30 minutes before serving.

Nutrition:

- Fat: 1g
- Carbohydrates: 40g
- Fiber: 5g
- Protein: 4g

24. Mini Mac in a Bowl

Preparation Time: 5 Minutes
Cooking Time: 15 Minutes
Servings: 1
Ingredients:

- 5 Ounces of lean ground beef
- 2 Tablespoons of diced white or yellow onion.
- 1/8 Teaspoon of onion powder
- 1/8 Teaspoon of white vinegar
- 1 Ounce of dill pickle slices
- 1 Teaspoon sesame seed
- 3 Cups of shredded romaine lettuce
- Cooking spray
- 2 Tablespoons reduced-fat shredded cheddar cheese
- 2 Tablespoons of wish-bone light thousand island as dressing

Directions:

1. Place a lightly greased small skillet on fire to heat.
2. Add your onion to cook for about 2-3 minutes.
3. Next, add the beef and allow cooking until it's brown.
4. Next, mix your vinegar and onion powder with the dressing.
5. Finally, top the lettuce with the cooked meat and sprinkle cheese on it; add your pickle slices.
6. Drizzle the mixture with the sauce and sprinkle the sesame seeds.
7. Your mini mac in a bowl is ready to eat.

Nutrition:

- Calories: 150
- Protein: 21g
- Carbohydrates: 32g
- Fats: 19g

25. Mini Zucchini Bites

Preparation Time: 10 Minutes
Cooking Time: 10 Minutes
Servings: 6
Ingredients:

- 1 Zucchini, cut into thick circles
- 3 Cherry tomatoes, halved
- ½ Cup parmesan cheese, grated
- Salt and pepper to taste
- 1 Tsp. Chives, chopped

Directions:

1. Preheat the oven to 390 degrees F.
2. Add wax paper to a baking sheet.
3. Arrange the zucchini pieces.
4. Add the cherry halves to each zucchini slice.
5. Add parmesan cheese, chives, and sprinkle with salt and pepper.
6. Bake for 10 minutes. Serve.

Nutrition:

- Fat: 1.0g
- Cholesterol: 5.0mg
- Sodium: 400.3mg
- Potassium: 50.5mg
- Carbohydrates: 7.3g

26. Lean and Green Smoothie 2

Preparation Time: 5 Minutes
Cooking Time: 0 Minutes
Servings: 1
Ingredients:

- Six kale leaves
- Two peeled oranges
- 2 Cups of mango kombucha
- 2 Cups of chopped pineapple
- 2 Cups of water

Directions:

1. Break up the oranges, place them in the blender.
2. Add the mango kombucha, chopped pineapple, and kale leaves into the blender.
3. Blend everything until it is smooth.
4. Smoothie is ready to be taken.

Nutrition:

- Calories: 81
- Protein: 2g
- Carbohydrates: 19g
- Fats: 1g

27. Mushroom & Spinach Omelet

Preparation Time: 20 Minutes
Cooking Time: 20 Minutes
Servings: 3
Ingredients:

- 2 Tablespoons butter, divided
- 6-8 Fresh mushrooms, sliced, 5 ounces
- Chives, chopped, optional
- Salt and pepper, to taste
- 1 Handful baby spinach, about ½ ounce
- Pinch garlic powder
- 4 Eggs, beaten
- 1-ounce Shredded swiss cheese

Directions:

1. In a very large saucepan, sauté the mushrooms in one tablespoon of butter until soft—season with salt, pepper, and garlic.
2. Remove the mushrooms from the pan and keep warm. Heat the remaining tablespoon of butter in the same skillet over medium heat.
3. Beat the eggs with a little salt and pepper and add to the hot butter. Turn the pan over to coat the entire bottom of the pan with the beaten eggs. Once the egg is almost done, place the cheese over the middle of the tortilla.
4. Fill the cheese with spinach leaves and hot mushrooms. Let cook for about a minute for the spinach to start to wilt. Fold the empty side of the tortilla carefully over the filling and slide it onto a plate and sprinkle with chives, if desired.
5. Alternatively, you can make two tortillas using half the mushroom, spinach, and cheese filling in each.

Nutrition:

- Calories: 321
- Fat: 26g
- Protein: 19g
- Carbohydrate: 4g
- Dietary Fiber: 1g

28. Whole-Wheat Blueberry Muffins

Preparation Time: 5 Minutes
Cooking Time: 25 Minutes
Servings: 8
Ingredients:

- ½ Cup plant-based milk
- ½ Cup unsweetened applesauce
- ½ Cup maple syrup
- 1 Teaspoon vanilla extract
- 2 Cups whole-wheat flour
- ½ Teaspoon baking soda
- 1 Cup blueberries

Directions:

1. Preheat the oven to 375°F.
2. In a large bowl, mix the milk, applesauce, maple syrup, and vanilla.
3. Stir in the flour and baking soda until no dry flour is left and the batter is smooth.
4. Gently fold in the blueberries until they are evenly distributed throughout the batter.
5. In a muffin tin, fill eight muffin cups with three-quarters full of batter.
6. Bake for 25 minutes, or until you can stick a knife into the center of a muffin and it comes out clean. Allow cooling before serving.

Tip: Both frozen and fresh blueberries will work great in this recipe. The only difference will be that muffins using fresh blueberries will cook slightly quicker than those using frozen.
Nutrition:

- Fat: 1g
- Carbohydrates: 45g
- Fiber: 2g
- Protein: 4g

29. Sweet Cashew Cheese Spread

Preparation Time: 5 Minutes
Cooking Time: 5 Minutes
Servings: 10 Servings
Ingredients:

- Stevia (5 drops)
- Cashews (2 cups, raw)
- Water (½ cup)

Directions:

1. Soak the cashews overnight in water.
2. Next, drain the excess water then transfer cashews to a food processor.
3. Add in the stevia and the water.
4. Process until smooth.
5. Serve chilled. Enjoy.

Nutrition:

- Fat: 7g
- Cholesterol: 0mg
- Sodium: 12.6mg
- Carbohydrates: 5.7g

30. Mouthwatering Tuna Melts

Preparation Time: 15 Minutes
Cooking TIme: 20 Minutes
Servings: 8
Ingredients:

- 1/8 Teaspoon Salt
- 1/3 Cup onion, chopped
- 16 1/3 Ounces Biscuits, refrigerated, flaky layers
- 10 Ounces Tuna, water-packed, drained
- 1/3 Cup Mayonnaise
- 1/8 Teaspoon Pepper
- 4 Ounces Cheddar cheese, shredded
- Tomato, chopped
- Sour cream
- Lettuce, shredded

Directions:

1. Preheat the air fryer at 325 degrees Fahrenheit.
2. Put some cooking spray onto a cookie sheet.
3. Mix tuna with mayonnaise, pepper, salt, and onion.
4. Separate the dough, so you have eight biscuits; press each into 5-inch rounds.
5. Arrange four biscuit rounds on the sheet. Fill at the center with tuna mixture before topping with cheese. Cover with the remaining biscuit rounds and press to seal.
6. Air-fry for fifteen to twenty minutes, slice each sandwich into halves. Serve each piece topped with lettuce, tomato, and sour cream.

Nutrition:

- Calories: 320
- Fat: 10g
- Protein: 10g
- Carbohydrates: 20g

31. Easiest Tuna Cobbler Ever

Preparation Time: 15 Minutes
Cooking Time: 25 Minutes
Servings: 4
Ingredients:

- Water, cold (1/3 cup)
- Tuna, canned, drained (10 ounces)
- Sweet pickle relish (2 tablespoons)
- Mixed vegetables, frozen (1 ½ cups)
- Soup, cream of chicken, condensed (10 ¾ ounces)
- Pimientos, sliced, drained (2 ounces)
- Lemon juice (1 teaspoon)
- Paprika

Directions:

1. Preheat the air fryer at 375 degrees Fahrenheit.
2. Mist cooking spray into a round casserole (1 ½ quart).
3. Mix the frozen vegetables with milk, soup, lemon juice, relish, pimientos, and tuna in a saucepan— cook for 8 minutes over medium heat.
4. Fill the casserole with the tuna mixture.
5. Combine the biscuit mix with cold water to form a soft dough. Beat for half a minute before pouring four spoonfuls into the casserole.
6. Dust the dish with paprika before air-frying for twenty to twenty-five minutes.

Nutrition:

- Calories: 320
- Fat: 10g
- Protein: 20g
- Carbohydrates: 30g

32. Lean and Green Smoothie 1

Preparation Time: 5 Minutes
Cooking Time: 0 Minutes
Servings: 1
Ingredients:

- 2 ½ Cups of kale leaves
- 3/4 Cup of chilled apple juice
- 1 Cup of cubed pineapple
- ½ Cup of frozen green grapes
- ½ Cup of chopped apple

Directions:

1. Place the pineapple, apple juice, apple, frozen green grapes, and kale leaves in a blender.
2. Cover and blend until it's smooth.
3. Smoothie is ready and can be garnished with halved grapes if you wish.

Nutrition:

- Calories: 81
- Protein: 2g
- Carbohydrates: 19g
- Fats: 1g

33. Deliciously Homemade Pork Buns

Preparation Time: 20 Minutes
Cooking Time: 25 Minutes
Servings: 8
Ingredients:

- 3 Pieces green onions, sliced thinly
- 1 Egg, beaten
- 1 Cup of pulled pork, diced, w/ barbecue sauce
- 16 1/3 Ounces buttermilk biscuits, refrigerated
- 1 Teaspoon soy sauce

Directions:

1. Preheat the air fryer at 325 degrees Fahrenheit.
2. Use parchment paper to line your baking sheet.
3. Combine pork with green onions.
4. Separate and press the dough to form 8 four-inch rounds.
5. Fill each biscuit round's center with two tablespoons of pork mixture. Cover with the dough edges and seal by pinching. Arrange the buns on the sheet and brush with a mixture of soy sauce and egg.
6. Cook in the air fryer for twenty to twenty-five minutes.

Nutrition:

- Calories: 240
- Fat: 0g
- Protein: 0g
- Carbohydrates: 20g

34. Yogurt Garlic Chicken

Preparation Time: 30 Minutes
Cooking Time: 60 Minutes
Servings: 6
Ingredients:

- 6 Pieces pita bread rounds, halved
- 1 Cup English cucumber, sliced thinly, w/ each slice halved

Chicken & vegetables:

- 3 Tablespoons olive oil
- ½ Teaspoon of black pepper, freshly ground
- 20 Ounces chicken thighs, skinless, boneless
- 1 Piece bell pepper, red, sliced into half-inch portions
- 4 Pieces garlic cloves, chopped finely
- ½ Teaspoon cumin, ground
- 1 Piece red onion, medium, sliced into half-inch wedges
- ½ Cup yogurt, plain, fat-free
- 2 Tablespoons lemon juice
- 1 ½ Teaspoons salt
- ½ Teaspoon red pepper flakes, crushed
- ½ Teaspoon allspice, ground
- 1 Piece bell pepper, yellow, sliced into half-inch portions

Yogurt sauce:

- 2 Tablespoons olive oil
- 1/4 Teaspoon salt
- 1 Tablespoon parsley, flat-leaf, chopped finely
- 1 Cup yogurt, plain, fat-free
- 1 Tablespoon lemon juice, fresh
- 1 Piece garlic clove, chopped finely

Directions:

1. Mix the yogurt (½ cup), garlic cloves (4 pieces), olive oil (1 tablespoon), salt (1 teaspoon), lemon juice (2 tablespoons), pepper (1/4 teaspoon), allspice, cumin, and pepper flakes. Stir in the chicken and coat well. Cover and marinate in the fridge for two hours.
2. Preheat the air fryer at 400 degrees Fahrenheit.
3. Grease a rimmed baking sheet (18x13-inch) with cooking spray.

4. Toss the bell peppers and onion with remaining olive oil (2 tablespoons), pepper (1/4 teaspoon), and salt (½ teaspoon).
5. Arrange veggies on the baking sheets left side and the marinated chicken thighs (drain first) on the right side—cook in the air fryer for twenty-five to thirty minutes.
6. Mix the yogurt sauce ingredients.
7. Slice air-fried chicken into half-inch strips.
8. Top each pita round with chicken strips, roasted veggies, cucumbers, and yogurt sauce.

Nutrition:

- Calories: 380
- Fat: 10g
- Protein: 20g
- Carbohydrates: 30g

35. Tuna Spinach Casserole

Preparation Time: 30 Minutes
Cooking Time: 25 Minutes
Servings: 8
Ingredients:

- 18 Ounces mushroom soup, creamy
- ½ Cup milk
- 12 Ounces white tuna, solid, in water, drained
- 8 Ounces crescent dinner rolls, refrigerated
- 8 Ounces egg noodles, wide, uncooked
- 8 Ounces cheddar cheese, shredded
- 9 Ounces spinach, chopped, frozen, thawed, drained
- 2 Teaspoons lemon peel grated

Directions:

1. Preheat the oven to 350 degrees Fahrenheit.
2. Put cooking spray onto a glass baking dish (11x7-inch).
3. Follow package directions in cooking and draining the noodles.
4. Stir the cheese (1 ½ cups) and soup together in a skillet heated on medium. Once cheese melts, stir in your noodles, milk, spinach, tuna, and lemon peel. Once bubbling, pour into the prepped dish.
5. Unroll the dough and sprinkle with remaining cheese (½ cup). Roll up dough and pinch at the edges to seal. Slice into eight portions and place over the tuna mixture.
6. Put all in the Air-fry mode for twenty to twenty-five minutes.

Nutrition:

- Calories: 400
- Fat: 10g
- Protein: 20g
- Carbohydrates: 30g

36. Lean and Green Chicken Pesto Pasta

Preparation Time: 5 Minutes
Cooking Time: 15 Minutes
Servings: 1
Ingredients:

- 3 Cups of raw kale leaves
- 2 Tbsp. of olive oil
- 2 Cups of fresh basil
- 1/4 teaspoon salt
- 3 Tbsp. Lemon juice
- Three garlic cloves
- 2 Cups of cooked chicken breast
- 1 Cup of baby spinach
- 6 Ounces of uncooked chicken pasta
- 3 Ounces of diced fresh mozzarella
- Basil leaves or red pepper flakes to garnish

Directions:

1. Start by making the pesto; add the kale, lemon juice, basil, garlic cloves, olive oil, and salt to a blender and blend until smooth.
2. Add salt and pepper to taste.
3. Cook the pasta and strain off the water. Reserve 1/4 cup of the liquid.
4. Get a bowl and mix everything, the cooked pasta, pesto, diced chicken, spinach, mozzarella, and the reserved pasta liquid.
5. Sprinkle the mixture with additional chopped basil or red paper flakes (optional).
6. Now your salad is ready. You may serve it warm or chilled. Also, it can be taken as a salad mix-ins or as a side dish. Leftovers should be stored in the refrigerator inside an air-tight container for 3-5 days.

Nutrition:

- Calories: 244
- Protein: 20.5g
- Carbohydrates: 22.5g
- Fats: 10g

37. Open-Face Egg Sandwiches With Cilantro-Jalapeño Spread

Preparation Time: 20 Minutes
Cooking Time: 10 Minutes
Servings: 2
Ingredients:
For the cilantro and jalapeño spread:

- 1 Cup filled up fresh cilantro leaves and stems (about a bunch)
- 1 Jalapeño pepper, seeded and roughly chopped
- ½ Cup extra-virgin olive oil
- ¼ Cup pepitas (hulled pumpkin seeds), raw or roasted
- 2 Garlic cloves, thinly sliced
- 1 Tablespoon freshly squeezed lime juice
- 1 Teaspoon kosher salt

For the eggs:

- 4 Large eggs
- ¼ Cup milk
- ¼ to ½ Teaspoon Kosher Salt
- 2 Tablespoons butter

For the sandwich:

- 2 Bread slices
- 1 Tablespoon butter
- 1 Avocado, halved, pitted, and divided into slices
- Microgreens or sprouts for garnish

Directions:
To make the cilantro and jalapeño spread:

1. In a food processor, combine the cilantro, jalapeño, oil, pepitas, garlic, lime juice, and salt. Whirl until smooth. Refrigerate it if preparing in advance; otherwise, set it aside.

To make the eggs:

1. In a medium bowl, whisk the eggs, milk, and salt.
2. Dissolve the butter in a skillet over low heat, swirling to coat the bottom of the pan. Pour in the whisked eggs.
3. Cook until they begin to set, using a heatproof spatula, push them to the sides, allowing the uncooked portions to run into the bottom of the skillet.

4. Continue until the eggs are set.

To assemble the sandwiches:

1. Toast the bread and spread it with butter.
2. Spread a spoonful of the cilantro-jalapeño spread on each piece of toast. Top each with scrambled eggs.
3. Arrange avocado over each sandwich and garnish with microgreens.

Nutrition:

- Calories: 711
- Total fat: 4g
- Cholesterol: 54mg
- Fiber: 12g
- Protein: 12g
- Sodium: 327mg

38. Lemony Parmesan Salmon

Preparation Time: 10 Minutes
Cooking Time: 25 Minutes
Servings: 4
Ingredients:

- 2 Tablespoons butter, melted
- 2 Tablespoons green onions, sliced thinly
- 3/4 Cups breadcrumbs, white, fresh
- 1/4 Teaspoon thyme leaves, dried
- 1 Piece salmon fillet, 1 ¼-pound
- 1/4 Teaspoon salt
- 1/4 Cup parmesan cheese, grated
- 2 Teaspoons lemon peel, grated

Directions:

1. Preheat the oven to 350 degrees Fahrenheit.
2. Mist cooking spray onto a baking pan (shallow). Fill with pat-dried salmon—brush salmon with butter (1 tablespoon) before sprinkling with salt.
3. Combine the breadcrumbs with onions, thyme, lemon peel, cheese, and remaining butter (1 tablespoon).
4. Cover salmon with the breadcrumb mixture. Air-fry for fifteen to twenty-five minutes.

Nutrition:

- Calories: 290
- Fat: 10g
- Protein: 30g
- Carbohydrates: 0g

39. Chicken Omelet

Preparation Time: 5 Minutes
Cooking Time: 15 Minutes
Servings: 1
Ingredients:

- 2 Bacon slices; cooked and crumbled
- 2 Eggs
- 1 Tablespoon homemade mayonnaise
- 1 Tomato; chopped.
- 1-Ounce rotisserie chicken; shredded
- 1 Teaspoon mustard
- 1 Small avocado; pitted, peeled, and chopped.
- Salt and black pepper, to the taste.

Directions:

1. In a bowl, mix eggs with some salt and pepper and whisk gently.
2. Heat up a pan over medium heat; spray with some cooking oil, add eggs and cook your omelet for 5 minutes
3. Add chicken, avocado, tomato, bacon, mayo, and mustard on one half of the omelet.
4. Fold omelet, cover the pan and cook for 5 minutes more
5. Transfer to a plate and serve

Nutrition:

- Calories: 400
- Fat: 32
- Fiber: 6
- Carbs: 4
- Protein: 25

40. Pepper Pesto Lamb

Preparation Time: 15 Minutes
Cooking Time: 1 Hour 15 Minutes
Servings: 12
Ingredients:
For the Pesto:

- 1/4 Cup rosemary leaves, fresh
- 3 Pieces garlic cloves
- 3/4 Cups parsley, fresh, packed firmly
- 1/4 Cup mint leaves, fresh
- 2 Tablespoons olive oil

Lamb:

- 7 ½ Ounces red bell peppers, roasted, drained
- 5 Pounds leg of lamb, boneless, rolled
- 2 Teaspoons seasoning, lemon pepper

Directions:

1. Preheat the oven to 325 degrees Fahrenheit.
2. Mix the pesto ingredients in the food processor.
3. Unroll the lamb and cover the cut side with pesto. Top with roasted peppers before rolling up the lamb and tying with kitchen twine.
4. Coat lamb with seasoning (lemon pepper) and air-fry for one hour.

Nutrition:

- Calories: 310
- Fat: 10g
- Protein: 40.0g
- Carbohydrates: 0g

41. Best Whole Wheat Pancakes

Preparation Time: 10 Minutes
Cooking Time: 20 Minutes
Servings: 1
Ingredients:

- 3/4 Tablespoons ground flaxseed
- 2 Tablespoons warm water
- ½ Cups whole wheat pastry flour
- 1/8 Cup rye flour
- ½ Tablespoons double-acting baking powder
- 1/4 Teaspoon ground cinnamon
- 1/8 Teaspoon ground ginger
- 1 Cup unsweetened nondairy milk
- 3/4 Tablespoons pure maple syrup
- 1/4 Teaspoon vanilla extract

Directions:

1. Mix the warm water and flaxseed in a large bowl. Set aside for at least 5 minutes.
2. Whisk together the pastry and rye flours, baking powder, cinnamon, and ginger.
3. Whisk together the milk, maple syrup, and vanilla in a large bowl. Make use of a spatula, fold the wet ingredients into the dry ingredients. Fold in the soaked flaxseed until fully incorporated.
4. Heat a large skillet or nonstick griddle over medium-high heat.
5. Working in batches, three to four pancakes at a time, add 1/4-cup portions of batter to the hot skillet.
6. Cook for 3 to 4 minutes on each side until golden brown or no liquid batter is visible.

Nutrition:

- Calories: 301
- Fat: 4g
- Protein: 10g
- Carbohydrates: 57g
- Fiber: 10g

42. Spiced Pumpkin Muffins

Preparation Time: 15 Minutes
Cooking Time: 20 Minutes
Servings: 1
Ingredients:

- 1/6 Tablespoons ground flaxseed
- ¼4 Cup of water
- 1/8 Cups whole wheat flour
- 1/6 Teaspoons baking powder
- 5/6 Teaspoons ground cinnamon
- 1/12 Teaspoon baking soda
- 1/12 Teaspoon ground ginger
- 1/16 Teaspoon ground nutmeg
- 1/32 Teaspoon ground cloves
- 1/6 Cup pumpkin puree
- 1/12 Cup pure maple syrup
- ¼4 Cup unsweetened applesauce
- ¼4 Cup unsweetened nondairy milk
- ½ Teaspoons vanilla extract

Directions:

1. Preheat the oven to 350°F. Line a 12-cup metal muffin pan with parchment paper liners, or use a silicone muffin pan.
2. First, mix the flaxseed and water in a large bowl, then keep it aside.
3. In a medium bowl, stir together the flour, baking powder, cinnamon, baking soda, ginger, nutmeg, and cloves.
4. In a medium bowl, stir up the maple syrup, pumpkin puree, applesauce, milk, and vanilla. Pour the wet ingredients into the dry ingredients making use of a spatula.
5. Fold the soaked flaxseed into the batter until evenly combined, but do not over mix the batter, or your muffins will become dense. Spoon about 1/4 cup of batter per muffin into your prepared muffin pan.
6. Bake for 18 to 20 minutes, or until a toothpick inserted into the center of a muffin comes out clean. Remove the muffins from the pan.
7. Transfer to a wire rack for cooling.
8. Store in an airtight container that is at room temperature.

Nutrition:

- Calories: 115
- Fat: 1g
- Protein: 3g
- Carbohydrates: 25g
- Fiber: 3g

Chapter 4. Salads

43. Blueberry Cantaloupe Avocado Salad

Preparation Time: 5 Minutes
Cooking Time: 0 Minutes
Servings: 2
Ingredients:

- 1 Diced cantaloupe
- 2–3 Chopped avocados
- 1 Package of blueberries
- ¼ Cup olive oil
- 1/8 Cup balsamic vinegar

Directions:

1. Mix all ingredients.

Nutrition:

- Calories: 406
- Protein: 9g
- Carbohydrate: 32g
- Fat: 5g

44. Wild Rice Prawn Salad

Preparation Time: 5 Minutes
Cooking Time: 35 Minutes
Servings: 6
Ingredients:

- ¾ Cup wild rice
- 1¾ Cups chicken stock
- 1 Pound prawns
- Salt and pepper to taste
- 2 Tablespoons lemon juice
- 2 Tablespoons extra virgin olive oil
- 2 Cups arugula

Directions:

1. Combine the rice and chicken stock in a saucepan and cook until the liquid has been absorbed entirely.
2. Transfer the rice to a salad bowl.
3. Season the prawns with salt and pepper and drizzle them with lemon juice and oil.
4. Heat a grill pan over a medium flame.
5. Place the prawns on the hot pan and cook on each side for 2-3 minutes.
6. For the salad, combine the rice with arugula and prawns and mix well.
7. Serve the salad fresh.

Nutrition:

- Calories: 207
- Fat: 4g
- Protein: 20.6g
- Carbohydrates: 17g

45. Beet Salad (from Israel)

Preparation Time: 5 Minutes
Cooking Time: 0 Minutes
Servings: 2
Ingredients:

- 2–3 Fresh, raw beets grated or shredded in food processor
- 3 Tablespoons olive oil
- 2 Tablespoons balsamic vinegar
- ¼ Teaspoon salt
- 1/3 Teaspoon cumin
- Dash stevia powder or liquid
- Dash pepper

Directions:

1. Mix all ingredients together for the best raw beet salad.

Nutrition:

- Calories: 156
- Protein: 8g
- Carbohydrate: 40g
- Fat: 5g

46. Greek Salad

Preparation Time: 15 Minutes
Cooking Time: 15 Minutes
Servings: 5
Ingredients:
For the Dressing:

- ½ Teaspoon black pepper
- ¼ Teaspoon salt
- ½ Teaspoon oregano
- 1 Tablespoon garlic powder
- 2 Tablespoons Balsamic
- 1/3 Cup olive oil

For the Salad:

- ½ Cup sliced black olives
- ½ Cup chopped parsley, fresh
- 1 Small red onion, thin-sliced
- 1 Cup cherry tomatoes, sliced
- 1 Bell pepper, yellow, chunked
- 1 Cucumber, peeled, quartered, and sliced
- 4 Cups chopped romaine lettuce
- ½ Teaspoon salt
- 2 Tablespoons olive oil

Directions:

1. In a small bowl, blend all of the ingredients for the dressing and let this set in the refrigerator while you make the salad.
2. To assemble the salad, mix together all the ingredients in a large-sized bowl and toss the veggies gently but thoroughly to mix.
3. Serve the salad with the dressing in amounts as desired

Nutrition:

- Calories: 234
- Fat: 16.1g
- Protein: 5g
- Carbs: 48g

47. Norwegian Niçoise Salad Smoked Salmon Cucumber Egg and Asparagus

Preparation Time: 20 Minutes
Cooking Time: 5 Minutes
Servings: 4
Ingredients:
For the vinaigrette:

- 3 Tablespoons walnut oil
- 2 Tablespoons champagne vinegar
- 1 Tablespoon chopped fresh dill
- ½ Teaspoon kosher salt
- ¼ Teaspoon ground mustard
- Freshly ground black pepper

For the salad:

- Handful green beans, trimmed
- 1 (3- to 4-ounce) Package spring greens
- 12 Spears pickled asparagus
- 4 Large soft-boiled eggs, halved
- 8 Ounces smoked salmon, thinly sliced
- 1 Cucumber, thinly sliced
- 1 Lemon, quartered

Directions:

1. To make the dressing. In a small bowl, whisk the oil, vinegar, dill, salt, ground mustard, and a few grinds of pepper until emulsified. Set aside.
2. To make the salad. Start by blanching the green beans, bring a pot of salted water to a boil. Drop in the beans. Cook for 1 to 2 minutes until they turn bright green, then immediately drain and rinse under cold water. Set aside.
3. Divide the spring greens among four plates. Toss each serving with dressing to taste. Arrange three asparagus spears, one egg, 2 ounces of salmon, one-fourth of the cucumber slices, and a lemon wedge on each plate. Serve immediately.

Nutrition:

- Calories: 257
- Total fat: 18g
- Total carbs: 6g
- Cholesterol: 199mg
- Fiber: 2g
- Protein: 19g
- Sodium: 603mg

48. Mediterranean Chickpea Salad

Preparation Time: 5 Minutes
Cooking Time: 20 Minutes
Servings: 6
Ingredients:

- 1 Can chickpeas, drained
- 1 Fennel bulb, sliced
- 1 Red onion, sliced
- 1 Teaspoon dried basil
- 1 Teaspoon dried oregano
- 2 Tablespoons chopped parsley
- 4 Garlic cloves, minced
- 2 Tablespoons lemon juice
- 2 Tablespoons extra virgin olive oil
- Salt and pepper to taste

Directions:

1. Combine the chickpeas, fennel, red onion, herbs, garlic, lemon juice, and oil in a salad bowl.
2. Add salt and pepper and serve the salad fresh.

Nutrition:

- Calories: 200
- Fat: 9g
- Protein: 4g
- Carbohydrates: 28g

49. Romaine Lettuce and Radicchios Mix

Preparation Time: 6 Minutes
Cooking Time: 0 Minutes
Servings: 4
Ingredients:

- 2 Tablespoons olive oil
- A pinch of salt and black pepper
- 2 Spring onions, chopped
- 3 Tablespoons Dijon mustard
- Juice of 1 lime
- ½ Cup basil, chopped
- 4 Cups romaine lettuce heads, chopped
- 3 Radicchios, sliced

Directions:

1. In a salad bowl, mix the lettuce with the spring onions and the other ingredients, toss and serve.

Nutrition:

- Calories: 87
- Fats: 2g
- Fiber: 1g
- Carbs: 1g
- Protein: 2g

50. Chicken Broccoli Salad With Avocado Dressing

Preparation Time: 5 Minutes
Cooking Time: 40 Minutes
Servings: 6
Ingredients:

- 2 Chicken breasts
- 1 Pound broccoli, cut into florets
- 1 Avocado, peeled and pitted
- ½ Lemon, juiced
- 2 Garlic cloves
- ¼ Teaspoon chili powder
- ¼ Teaspoon cumin powder
- Salt and pepper to taste

Directions:

1. Cook the chicken in a large pot of salty water.
2. Drain and cut the chicken into small cubes—place in a salad bowl.
3. Add the broccoli and mix well.
4. Combine the avocado, lemon juice, garlic, chili powder, cumin powder, salt, and pepper in a blender. Pulse until smooth.
5. Spoon the dressing over the salad and mix well.
6. Serve the salad fresh.

Nutrition:

- Calories: 195
- Fat: 11g
- Protein: 14g
- Carbohydrates: 3g

51. Zucchini Salmon Salad

Preparation Time: 5 Minutes
Cooking Time: 10 Minutes
Servings: 3
Ingredients:

- 2 Salmon fillets
- 2 Tablespoons soy sauce
- 2 Zucchinis, sliced
- Salt and pepper to taste
- 2 Tablespoons extra virgin olive oil
- 2 Tablespoons sesame seeds

Directions:

1. Drizzle the salmon with soy sauce.
2. Heat a grill pan over a medium flame. Cook salmon on the grill on each side for 2-3 minutes.
3. Season the zucchini with salt and pepper and place it on the grill as well. Cook on each side until golden.
4. Place the zucchini, salmon, and the rest of the ingredients in a bowl.
5. Serve the salad fresh.

Nutrition:

- Calories: 224
- Fat: 19g
- Protein: 18g
- Carbohydrates: 0g

52. Warm Chorizo Chickpea Salad

Preparation Time: 5 Minutes
Cooking Time: 20 Minutes
Servings: 6
Ingredients:

- 1 Tablespoon extra-virgin olive oil
- 4 Chorizo links, sliced
- 1 Red onion, sliced
- 4 Roasted red bell peppers, chopped
- 1 Can chickpeas, drained
- 2 Cups cherry tomatoes
- 2 Tablespoons balsamic vinegar
- Salt and pepper to taste

Directions:

1. Heat the oil in a skillet and add the chorizo. Cook briefly just until fragrant, then add the onion, bell peppers, and chickpeas and cook for two additional minutes.
2. Transfer the mixture to a salad bowl, then add the tomatoes, vinegar, salt, and pepper.
3. Mix well and serve the salad right away.

Nutrition:

- Calories: 359
- Fat: 18g
- Protein: 15g
- Carbohydrates: 21g

53. Broccoli Salad

Preparation Time: 5 Minutes
Cooking Time: 0 Minutes
Servings: 2
Ingredients:

- 1 Head broccoli, chopped
- 2–3 Slices of fried bacon, crumbled
- 1 Diced green onion
- ½ Cup raisins or craisins
- ½–1 Cup of chopped pecans
- ¾ Cups sunflower seeds
- ½ Cup of pomegranate

Dressing:

- 1 Cup Organic Mayonnaise
- ¼ Cup Baking Stevia
- 2 Teaspoons White Vinegar

Directions:

1. Mix all ingredients together. Mix dressing and fold into the salad.

Nutrition:

- Calories: 239
- Protein: 10g
- Carbohydrate: 33g
  Fat: 2g

Chapter 5. Soup and Stew Recipes

54. Roasted Tomato Soup

Difficulty: Easy
Preparation Time: 20 Minutes
Cooking Time: 50 Minutes
Servings: 6
Ingredients:

- 3 Pounds of tomatoes, halved (1green)
- 6 Garlic(smashed) (½ condiment)
- 4 Teaspoons of cooking oil or virgin oil (1/8 condiment)
- Salt to taste (1/8 condiment)
- 1/4 Cup of heavy cream (optional) (½ healthy fat)
- Sliced fresh basil leaves for garnish (1/8green)

Directions:

1. Set the oven at medium heat of about 427°F and let it preheat
2. In your mixing bowl, mix the halved tomatoes, garlic, olive oil, salt, and pepper
3. Spread the tomato mixture on the already prepared baking sheet
4. For a process of 20- 28 minutes, roast and stir
5. Then remove it from the oven, and the roasted vegetables should now be transferred to a soup pot
6. Stir in the basil leaves
7. Blend in small portions in a blender
8. Serve immediately

Nutrition:

- Fat: 5.9g
- Protein: 2.3g
- Calories: 126

55. Lemon-Garlic Chicken

Difficulty: Average
Preparation Time: 5 Minutes
Cooking Time: 45 Minutes
Servings: 4
Ingredients:

- 1 Small lemon, juiced (1/8 condiment)
- 1 3/4 lb. of bone-in, skinless chicken thighs (1 lean)
- 2 Tablespoons of fresh oregano, minced (1/8green)
- 2 Cloves of garlic, minced (1/8 condiment)
- 2 lbs. of asparagus, trimmed (1/8green)
- 1/4 Teaspoon each or less for black pepper and salt (1/8 condiment)

Directions:

1. Preheat the oven to about 350°F. Put the chicken in a medium-sized bowl.
2. Now, add the garlic, oregano, lemon juice, pepper, and salt and toss together to combine.
3. Roast for 40 minutes.
4. Once the chicken thighs have been cooked, remove and keep them aside to rest.
5. Now, steam the asparagus on a stovetop or in a microwave to the desired doneness.
6. Serve asparagus with roasted chicken thighs.

Nutrition:

- Calories: 350
- Fat: 10g
- Protein: 32g

56. Quick Lentil Chili

Difficulty: Easy
Preparation Time: 15 Minutes
Cooking Time: 1 Hour and 20 Minutes
Servings: 10
Ingredients:

- 1½ Cups of seeded or diced pepper (1green)
- 5 Cups of vegetable broth (it should have a low sodium content) (1 condiment)
- 1 Tablespoon of garlic (1/8 condiment)
- 1/4 Teaspoon of freshly ground pepper (1/8 condiment)
- 1 Cup of red lentils (1/4green)
- 3 Filled teaspoons of chili powder (1/8 condiment)
- 1 Tablespoon of grounded cumin (1/8 condiment)

Directions:

1. Place your pot over medium heat
2. Combine your onions, red peppers, low sodium vegetable broth, garlic, salt, and pepper
3. Cook and always stir until the onions are more translucent and all the liquid evaporated. This will take about 10mins.
4. Add the remaining broth, lime juice, chili powder, lentils, cumin, and boil.
5. Reduce heat at this point, cover it for about 15 minutes to simmer until the lentils are appropriately cooked
6. Drizzle a little water if the mixture seems to be thick.
7. The chili will be appropriately done when most of the water is absorbed.
8. Serve and enjoy.

Nutrition:

- Protein: 2.3g
- Calories: 121
- Fat: 2.9g

57. Creamy Cauliflower Soup

Difficulty: Average
Preparation Time: 15 Minutes
Cooking Time: 30 Minutes
Servings: 6
Ingredients:

- 5 Cups cauliflower rice (1green)
- 8 oz. Cheddar cheese, grated (1 healthy fat)
- 2 Cups unsweetened almond milk (½ healthy fat)
- 2 Cups vegetable stock (1 condiment)
- 2 Tbsp. water (½ condiment)
- 2 Garlic cloves, minced (1/4 condiment)
- 1 Tbsp. olive oil (1/8 condiment)

Directions:

1. Cook olive oil in a large stockpot over medium heat.
2. Add garlic and cook for 1-2 minutes. Add cauliflower rice and water.
3. Cover and cook for 5-7 minutes.
4. Now add vegetable stock and almond milk and stir well.
5. Bring to a boil.
6. Turn heat to low and simmer for 5 minutes.
7. Turn off the heat.
8. Slowly add cheddar cheese and stir until smooth.
9. Season soup with pepper and salt.
10. Stir well and serve hot.

Nutrition:

- Calories: 214
- Fat: 16.5g
- Protein: 11.6g

58. Crackpot Chicken Taco Soup

Difficulty: Average
Preparation Time: 15 Minutes
Cooking Time: 6 Hours
Servings: 6
Ingredients:

- 2 Frozen boneless chicken breasts (1 lean)
- 2 Cans of white beans or black beans (1 healthy fat)
- 1 Can of diced tomatoes (1 healthy fat)
- ½ Packet of taco seasoning (1/8 condiment)
- ½ Teaspoon of Garlic salt (1/8 condiment)
- 1 Cup of chicken broth (1 condiment)
- Salt and pepper to taste (1/8 condiment)
  Tortilla chips, sour cream cheese, and cilantro as toppings (1
- healthy fat)

Directions:

1. Put your frozen chicken into the crockpot and place the other ingredients into the pool too.
2. Leave to cook for about 6-8 hours.
3. After cooking, take out the chicken and shred it to the size you want.
4. Finally, place the shredded chicken into the crockpot and put it on a slow cooker. Stir and allow to cook.
5. You can add more beans and tomatoes also to help stretch the meat and make it tastier.

Nutrition:

- Protein: 29g
- Fat: 4g
- Calories: 171

59. Cheeseburger Soup

Difficulty: Average
Preparation Time: 15 Minutes
Cooking Time: 45 Minutes
Servings: 4
Ingredients:

- 1 14.5 oz. can diced tomato (1green)
- 1 lb. of 90% lean ground beef (1 lean)
- 3/4 Cup of chopped celery (½ green)
- 2 Teaspoons of Worcestershire sauce (1/8 condiment)
- 3 Cups of low sodium chicken broth (1 condiment)
- 1/4 Teaspoon of salt (1/8 condiment)
- 1 Teaspoon of dried parsley (1/8green)
- 7 Cups of baby spinach (1green)
- 1/4 Teaspoon of ground pepper (1/8 condiment)
- 4 oz. of reduced-fat shredded cheddar cheese (½ healthy fat)

Directions:

1. Get a large soup pot and cook the beef until it becomes brown.
2. Add the celery and sauté until it becomes tender.
3. Remove from the heat and drain excess liquid. Stir in the broth, tomatoes, parsley, Worcestershire sauce, pepper, and salt.
4. Cover with the lid and allow it to simmer on low heat for about 20 minutes.
5. Add spinach and leave it to cook until it becomes wilted in about 1-3 minutes.
6. Top each of your servings with 1 ounce of cheese.

Nutrition:

- Calories: 400
- Protein: 44g
- Fat: 20g

60. Mushroom & Jalapeño Stew

Difficulty: Easy
Preparation Time: 20 Minutes
Cooking Time: 50 Minutes
Servings: 4
Ingredients:

- 2 Tsp. olive oil (1/8 condiment)
- 1 Cup leeks, chopped (½ green)
- 1 Garlic clove, minced (1/8 condiment)
- ½ Cup celery stalks, chopped (½ green)
- ½ Cup carrots, chopped (½ green)
- 1 Green bell pepper, chopped (½ green)
- 1 Jalapeño pepper, chopped (1/4green)
- 2 ½ Cups mushrooms, sliced (1 healthy fat)
- 1 ½ Cups vegetable stock (1 condiment)
- 2 Tomatoes, chopped (1green)
- 2 Thyme sprigs, chopped (1/4green)
- 1 Rosemary sprig, chopped (1/4green)
- 2 Bay leaves (1/4green)
- ½ Tsp. salt (1/8 condiment)
- 1/4 Tsp. ground black pepper (1/8 condiment)
- 2 Tbsp. vinegar (1/8 condiment)

Directions:

1. Set a pot over medium heat and warm oil.
2. Add in garlic and leeks and sauté until soft and translucent.
3. Add in the black pepper, celery, mushrooms, and carrots.
4. Cook as you stir for 12 minutes; stir in a splash of vegetable stock to ensure there is no sticking.
5. Stir in the rest of the ingredients.
6. Set heat to medium; allow to simmer for 25 to 35 minutes or until cooked through.
7. Divide into individual bowls and serve warm.

Nutrition:

- Calories: 65
- Fats: 2.7g
- Protein: 2.7g

61. Easy Cauliflower Soup

Difficulty: Easy
Preparation Time: 5 Minutes
Cooking Time: 15 Minutes
Servings: 4
Ingredients:

- 2 Tbsp. olive oil (1/4 condiment)
- 1 Tsp. garlic, minced (1/4 condiment)
- 1-pound cauliflower, cut into florets (1green)
- 1 Cup kale, chopped (½ green)
- 4 Cups vegetable broth (1 condiment)
- ½ Cup almond milk (½ healthy fat)
- ½ Tsp. salt (1/8 condiment)
- ½ Tsp. red pepper flakes (1/8 condiment)
- 1 Tbsp. fresh chopped parsley (1/4green)

Directions:

1. Set a pot over medium heat and warm the oil.
2. Add garlic and onions and sauté until browned and softened.
3. Place in vegetable broth, kale, and cauliflower; cook for 10 minutes until the mixture boils.
4. Stir in the pepper flakes, salt, and almond milk; reduce the heat and simmer the soup for 5 minutes.
5. Transfer the soup to an immersion blender and blend to achieve the desired consistency; top with parsley and serve immediately.

Nutrition:

- Calories: 172
- Fats: 10.3g
- Protein: 8.1g

62. Tofu Stir Fry With Asparagus Stew

Difficulty: Average
Preparation Time: 15 Minutes
Cooking Time: 30 Minutes
Servings: 4
Ingredients:

- 1-pound Asparagus, cut off stems (1green)
- 2 Tbsp. olive oil (1/8 condiment)
- 2 Blocks tofu, pressed and cubed (1 lean)
- 2 Garlic cloves, minced (1/8 condiment)
- 1 Tsp. Cajun spice mix (1/8 condiment)
- 1 Tsp. mustard (1/8 condiment)
- 1 Bell pepper, chopped (1/4green)
- 1/4 Cup vegetable broth (1green)
- Salt and black pepper, to taste (1/8 condiment)

Directions:

1. Using a huge saucepan with lightly salted water, place in asparagus and cook until tender for 10 minutes; drain.
2. Set a wok over high heat and warm olive oil; stir in tofu cubes and cook for 6 minutes.
3. Place in garlic and cook for 30 seconds until soft.
4. Stir in the remaining ingredients, including reserved asparagus, and cook for four more minutes.
5. Divide among plates and serve.

Nutrition:

- Calories: 138
- Fat: 8.9g
- Protein: 6.4g

63. Cream of Thyme Tomato Soup

Difficulty: Easy
Preparation Time: 5 Minutes
Cooking Time: 20 Minutes
Servings: 6
Ingredients:

- 2 Tbsp. ghee (½ healthy fat)
- ½ Cup raw cashew nuts, diced (½ healthy fat)
- 2 (28 oz.) Cans tomatoes (1green)
- 1 Tsp. fresh thyme leaves + extra to garnish (1/4green)
- 1 ½ Cups water (½ healthy fat)
- Salt and black pepper to taste (1/8 condiment)

Directions:

1. Cook ghee in a pot over medium heat and sauté the onions for 4 minutes until softened.
2. Stir in the tomatoes, thyme, water, cashews, and season with salt and black pepper.
3. Cover and bring to simmer for 10 minutes until thoroughly cooked.
4. Open, turn the heat off, and puree the ingredients with an immersion blender.
5. Adjust to taste and stir in the heavy cream.
6. Spoon into soup bowls and serve.

Nutrition:

- Calories: 310
- Fats: 27g
- Protein: 11g

64. Lime-Mint Soup

Difficulty: Difficult
Preparation Time: 5 Minutes
Cooking Time: 20 Minutes
Servings: 4
Ingredients:

- 4 Cups vegetable broth (1 condiment)
- 1/4 Cup fresh mint leaves (1/8 condiment)
- 1/4 Cup scallions (1/4green)
- 3 Garlic cloves, minced (1/8 condiment)
- 3 Tablespoons freshly squeezed lime juice (1/4 condiment)

Directions:

1. In a large stockpot, combine the broth, mint, scallions, garlic, and lime juice.
2. Bring to a boil over medium-high heat.
3. Cover, set heat to low, simmer for 15 minutes, and serve.

Nutrition:

- Fat: 2g
- Protein: 5g
- Calories: 214

Chapter 6. Vegan Recipes

65. Vegan Edamame Quinoa Collard Wraps

Preparation Time: 5 Minutes
Cooking Time: 15 Minutes
Servings: 4
Ingredients:
For the wrap:

- 2 to 3 Collard leaves
- 1/4 Cup Grated carrot
- 1/4 Cup Sliced cucumber
- 1/4 Thin strips Red bell pepper
- 1/4 Thin strips Orange bell pepper
- 1/3 Cup Cooked Quinoa
- 1/3 Cup Shelled defrosted edamame

For the dressing:

- 3 Tablespoons Fresh ginger root, peeled and chopped
- 1 Cup Cooked chickpeas
- 1 Garlic clove
- 4 Tablespoons Rice vinegar
- 2 Tablespoons Low sodium tamari/coconut aminos
- 2 Tablespoons Lime juice
- 1/4 Cup Water
- Few pinches of chili flakes
- 1 Stevia pack

Directions:

1. For the dressing, combine all the ingredients and purée in a food processor until smooth.
2. Load into a little jar or tub, and set aside.
3. Place the collar leaves on a flat surface, covering one another to create a tighter tie.
4. Take one tablespoon of ginger dressing and blend it up with the prepared quinoa.
5. Spoon the prepared quinoa onto the leaves and shape a simple horizontal line at the closest end.
6. Supplement the edamame with all the veggie fillings left over.
7. Drizzle around one tablespoon of the ginger dressing on top, then fold the cover's sides inwards.
8. Pullover the fillings, the side of the cover closest to you, then turn the whole body away to seal it up.

Nutrition:

- Calories: 295
- Sugar: 3g
- Sodium: 200mg
- Fat: 13g

66. Baked Cheesy Eggplant With Marinara

Preparation Time: 20 Minutes
Cooking Time: 45 Minutes
Servings: 3
Ingredients:

- 1 Clove garlic, sliced
- 1 Large eggplant
- 2 Tablespoons olive oil
- ½ Pinch salt, or as needed
- 1/4 Cup and 2 tablespoons dry bread crumbs
- 1/4 Cup and 2 tablespoons ricotta cheese
- 1/4 Cup grated Parmesan cheese
- 1/4 Cup water, plus more as needed
- 1/4 Teaspoon red pepper flakes
- 1-½ Cups prepared marinara sauce
- 1-½ Teaspoons olive oil
- 2 Tablespoons shredded pepper jack cheese
- Salt and freshly ground black pepper to taste

Directions:

1. Cut the eggplant crosswise into five pieces. Peel a pumpkin, grate it and cut it into two cubes.

2. Lightly turn skillet with one tablespoon olive oil. Heat the oil at 390°F for 5 minutes. Add half of the eggplants and cook for 2 minutes on each side. Transfer to a plate.
3. Add one tablespoon of olive oil and add garlic, cook for one minute. Add the chopped eggplants. Season with pepper flakes and salt. Cook for 4 minutes. Lower the heat to 330oF and continue cooking the eggplants until soft, about eight more minutes.
4. Stir in water and marinara sauce. Cook for 7 minutes until heated through. Stir every now and then. Transfer to a bowl.
5. In a bowl, whisk well pepper, salt, pepper jack cheese, Parmesan cheese, and ricotta. Evenly spread cheeses over eggplant strips and then fold in half.
6. Lay folded eggplant in baking pan. Pour the marinara sauce on top.
7. In a small bowl, whisk well olive oil and bread crumbs. Sprinkle all over the sauce.
8. Cook for 15 minutes at 390°F until tops are lightly browned.
9. Serve and enjoy.

Nutrition:

- Calories: 405
- Carbs: 41.1g
- Protein: 12.7g
- Fat: 21.4g

67. Creamy Spinach and Mushroom Lasagna

Preparation Time: 60 Minutes
Cooking Time: 20 Minutes
Servings: 6
Ingredients:

- 10 Lasagna noodles
- 1 Package whole milk ricotta
- 2 Packages of frozen chopped spinach.
- 4 Cups mozzarella cheese (divided and shredded)
- 3/4 Cups grated fresh Parmesan
- 3 Tablespoons chopped fresh parsley leaves (optional)

For the Sauce:

- 1/4 Cup of butter (unsalted)
- 2 Garlic cloves
- 1 Pound of thinly sliced cremini mushroom
- 1 Diced onion
- 1/4 Cup flour
- 4 Cups milk, kept at room temperature
- 1 Teaspoon basil (dried)
- Pinch of nutmeg
- Salt and freshly ground black pepper, to taste

Directions:

1. Preheat oven to 352 degrees F.
2. To make the sauce, over medium heat, melt your butter. Add garlic, mushrooms, and onion. Cook and stir at intervals until it becomes tender at about 3-4 minutes.
3. Whisk in flour until lightly browned; it takes about 1 minute for it to become brown.
4. Next, whisk in the milk gradually, and cook, constantly whisking, about 2-3 minutes till it becomes thickened. Stir in basil, oregano, and nutmeg, season with salt and pepper for taste.
5. Then set aside.
6. In another pot of boiling salted water, cook lasagna noodles according to the package instructions.
7. Spread one cup mushroom sauce onto the bottom of a baking dish; top it with four lasagna noodles, ½ of the spinach, one cup mozzarella cheese, and 1/4 cup Parmesan.
8. Repeat this process with the remaining noodles, mushroom sauce, and cheeses.

9. Place into oven and bake for 35-45 minutes, or until it starts bubbling. Then boil for 2-3 minutes until it becomes brown and translucent.
10. Let cool for 15 minutes.
11. Serve it with garnished parsley (optional)

Nutrition:

- Calories: 488.3 Cal
- Fats: 19.3g
- Cholesterol: 88.4mg
- Sodium: 451.9mg
- Carbohydrates: 51.0g
- Dietary Fiber: 7.0g
- Protein: 25.0g

68. Zucchini Parmesan Chips

Difficulty: Hard
Preparation Time: 5 Minutes
Cooking Time: 8 Minutes
Servings: 10
Ingredients:

- ½ Tsp. Paprika
- ½ C. Grated parmesan cheese
- ½ C. Italian breadcrumbs
- 1 Lightly beaten egg
- Thinly sliced zucchinis

Directions:

1. Use a very sharp knife or mandolin slicer to slice zucchini as thinly as you can—pat off extra moisture.
2. Beat the egg with a pinch of pepper and salt and a bit of water.
3. Combine paprika, cheese, and breadcrumbs in a bowl.
4. Dip slices of zucchini into the egg mixture and then into the breadcrumb mixture. Press gently to coat.
5. With olive oil or cooking spray, mist-coated zucchini slices, then place them into your air fryer in a single layer.
6. Cook 8 minutes at 350 degrees.
7. Sprinkle with salt and serve with salsa.

Nutrition:

- Calories: 211
- Fat: 16g
- Protein: 8g
- Sugar: 0g

69. Roasted Squash Puree

Preparation Time: 20 Minutes
Cooking Time: 6 to 7 Hours
Servings: 8
Ingredients:

- 1 (3-pound) Butternut squash, peeled, seeded, and cut into 1-inch pieces
- 3 (1-pound) Acorn squash, peeled, seeded, and cut into 1-inch pieces
- 2 Onions, chopped
- 3 Garlic cloves, minced
- 2 Tablespoons olive oil
- 1 Teaspoon dried marjoram leaves
- ½ Teaspoon salt
- 1/8 Teaspoon freshly ground black pepper

Directions:

1. In a 6-quart slow cooker, mix all of the ingredients.
2. Cover and cook on low for 6 to 7 hours or until the squash is tender when pierced with a fork.
3. Use a potato masher to mash the squash right in the slow cooker.

Nutrition:

- Calories: 175
- Carbohydrates: 38g
- Sugar: 1g
- Fiber: 3g
- Fat: 4g
- Saturated Fat: 1g
- Protein: 3g
- Sodium: 149mg

70. Air Fryer Brussels Sprouts

Difficulty: Hard
Preparation Time: 5 Minutes
Cooking Time: 10 Minutes
Servings: 5
Ingredients:

- ¼ Tsp. salt
- 1 Tbsp. balsamic vinegar
- 1 Tbsp. olive oil
- C. Brussels sprouts

Directions:

1. Cut Brussels sprouts in half lengthwise. Toss with salt, vinegar, and olive oil till coated thoroughly.
2. Add coated sprouts to the air fryer, cooking 8-10 minutes at 400 degrees. Shake after 5 minutes of cooking.
3. Brussels sprouts are ready to devour when brown and crisp!

Nutrition:

- Calories: 118
- Fat: 9g
- Protein: 11g
- Sugar: 1g

71. Thai Roasted Veggies

Preparation Time: 20 Minutes
Cooking Time: 6 to 8 Hours
Servings: 8
Ingredients:

- 4 Large carrots, peeled and cut into chunks
- 2 Onions, peeled and sliced
- 6 Garlic cloves, peeled and sliced
- 2 Parsnips, peeled and sliced
- 2 Jalapeño peppers, minced
- ½ Cup Roasted Vegetable Broth
- 1/3 Cup canned coconut milk
- 3 Tablespoons lime juice
- 2 Tablespoons grated fresh ginger root
- 2 Teaspoons curry powder

Directions:

1. In a 6-quart slow cooker, mix the carrots, onions, garlic, parsnips, and jalapeño peppers.
2. In a small bowl, mix the vegetable broth, coconut milk, lime juice, ginger root, and curry powder until well blended. Pour this mixture into the slow cooker.
3. Cover and cook on low for 6 to 8 hours, do it until the vegetables are tender when pierced with a fork.

Nutrition:

- Calories: 69
- Carbohydrates: 13g
- Sugar: 6g
- Fiber: 3g
- Fat: 3g
- Saturated Fat: 3g
- Protein: 1g
- Sodium: 95mg

72. Crispy Jalapeno Coins

Difficulty: Hard
Preparation Time: 10 Minutes
Cooking Time: 10 Minutes
Servings: 8 to 10
Ingredients:

- 1 Egg
- 2-3 Tbsp. coconut flour
- 1 Sliced and seeded jalapeno
- Pinch of garlic powder
- Pinch of onion powder
- Pinch of Cajun seasoning (optional)
- Pinch of pepper and salt

Directions:

1. Ensure your air fryer is preheated to 400 degrees.
2. Mix together all dry ingredients.
3. Pat jalapeno slices dry. Dip coins into the egg wash and then into the dry mixture. Toss to thoroughly coat.
4. Add coated jalapeno slices to the air fryer in a singular layer. Spray with olive oil.
5. Cook just till crispy.

Nutrition:

- Calories: 128
- Fat: 8g
- Protein: 7g
- Sugar: 0g

73. Crispy-Topped Baked Vegetables

Preparation Time: 10 Minutes
Cooking Time: 40 Minutes
Servings: 4
Ingredients:

- 2 Tbsp. Olive oil
- 1 Onion, chopped
- 1 Celery stalk, chopped
- 2 Carrots, grated
- ½-pound Turnips, sliced
- 1 Cup vegetable broth
- 1 Tsp. Turmeric
- Sea salt and black pepper, to taste
- ½ Tsp. Liquid smoke
- 1 Cup Parmesan cheese, shredded
- 2 Tbsp. Fresh chives, chopped

Directions:

1. Set oven to 360°F and grease a baking dish with olive oil.
2. Set a skillet over medium heat and warm olive oil.
3. Sweat the onion until soft, and place in the turnips, carrots, and celery; and cook for 4 minutes.
4. Remove the vegetable mixture from the baking dish.
5. Combine vegetable broth with turmeric, pepper, liquid smoke, and salt.
6. Spread this mixture over the vegetables.
7. Sprinkle with Parmesan cheese and bake for about 30 minutes.
8. Garnish with chives to serve.

Nutrition:

- Calories: 242 Cal
- Fats: 16.3g
- Carbohydrates: 8.6g
- Protein: 16.3g

74. Jicama Fries

Difficulty: Hard
Preparation Time: 10 Minutes
Cooking Time: 20 Minutes
Servings: 8
Ingredients:

- 1 Tbsp. Dried thyme
- ¾ C. Arrowroot flour
- ½ Large Jicama
- Eggs

Directions:

1. Sliced jicama into fries.
2. Whisk eggs together and pour over fries. Toss to coat.
3. Mix a pinch of salt, thyme, and arrowroot flour together. Toss egg-coated jicama into dry mixture, tossing to coat well.
4. Spray air fryer basket with olive oil and add fries—cook 20 minutes on the "CHIPS" setting. Toss halfway into the cooking process.

Nutrition:

- Calories: 211
- Fat: 19g
- Protein: 9g
- Sugar: 1g

75. Spaghetti Squash Tots

Difficulty: Hard
Preparation Time: 5 Minutes
Cooking Time: 15 Minutes
Servings: 8 to 10
Ingredients:

- ¼ Tsp. pepper
- ½ Tsp. salt
- 1 Thinly sliced scallion
- 1 Spaghetti squash

Directions:

1. Wash and cut the squash in half lengthwise. Scrap out the seeds.
2. With a fork, remove spaghetti meat by strands and throw out skins.
3. In a clean towel, toss in squash and wring out as much moisture as possible. Place in a bowl and with a knife, slice through meat a few times to cut up smaller.
4. Add pepper, salt, and scallions to squash and mix well.
5. Create "tot" shapes with your hands and place them in the air fryer. Spray with olive oil.
6. Cook 15 minutes at 350 degrees until golden and crispy!

Nutrition:

- Calories: 231
- Fat: 18g
- Protein: 5g
- Sugar: 0g

76. Low Carb Pork Dumplings With Dipping Sauce

Difficulty: Difficult
Preparation Time: 30 Minutes
Cooking Time: 20 Minutes
Servings: 6
Ingredients:

- 18 Dumpling wrappers (1 healthy fat)
- 1 Teaspoon olive oil (1/4 condiment)
- 4 Cups bok choy (chopped) (2 leans)
- 2 Tablespoons rice vinegar (½ condiment)
- 1 Tablespoon diced ginger (1/4 condiment)
- 1/4 Teaspoon crushed red pepper (½ green)
- 1 Tablespoon diced garlic (½ condiment)
- Lean ground pork ½ cup (2 leans)
- 2 Teaspoons Lite soy sauce (½ condiment)
- ½ Tsp. Honey (1/4 healthy fat)
- 1 Teaspoon Toasted sesame oil (1/4 condiment)
- Finely chopped scallions (1green)

Directions

1. In a large skillet, heat the olive oil, add the bok choy, cook for 6 minutes and add the garlic, ginger and cook for one minute. Transfer this mixture to a paper towel and pat dry any excess oil
2. In a bowl, add the mixture of bok choy, red pepper, and lean ground pork and mix well.
3. Place dumplings wrap on a plate and add a spoon to fill half of the wrapper. With water, seal the edges and fold them.
4. Spray air fryer basket with oil, add dumplings into the air fryer basket and cook at 375°F for 12 minutes or until golden brown.
5. Meanwhile, to make the sauce, combine the sesame oil, rice vinegar, shallot, soy sauce, and honey in a mixing bowl.
6. Serve the dumplings with the sauce.

Nutrition:

- Calories: 140
- Fat: 5g
- Protein: 12g

77. Gluten-Free Air Fryer Chicken Fried Brown Rice

Difficulty: Average
Preparation Time: 10 Minutes
Cooking Time: 20 Minutes
Servings: 2
Ingredients:

- 1 Cup Chicken Breast (1 lean)
- 1/4 Cup chopped White Onion (½ green)
- 1/4 Cup chopped Celery (½ green)
- 4 Cups Cooked brown rice (2 healthy fat)
- 1/4 Cup chopped Carrots (½ green)

Directions

1. Place the foil on the air fryer basket, make sure to leave room for airflow, roll up on the sides
2. Spray the film with olive oil. Mix all the ingredients.
3. On top of the foil, add all the ingredients to the air fryer basket.
4. Give a splash of olive oil to the mixture.
5. Cook for five minutes at 390°F.
6. Open the air fryer and give the mixture a spin
7. Cook for another five minutes at 390°F.
8. Remove from the air fryer and serve hot.

Nutrition

- Calories: 350
- Fat: 6g
- Protein: 22g

78. Air Fryer Cheesy Pork Chops

Difficulty: Average
Preparation Time: 5 Minutes
Cooking Time: 8 Minutes
Servings: 2
Ingredients:

- 2 Lean pork chops
- Half teaspoon of Salt (1/4 condiment)
- ½ Tsp. Garlic powder (1/4 condiment)
- 4 Tbsp. Shredded cheese (1 healthy fat)
- Chopped cilantro (1green)

Directions:

1. Let the air fryer preheat to 350 degrees.
2. With garlic, coriander and salt, rub the pork chops. Put the air fryer on. Let it cook for four minutes. Turn them over and then cook for extra two minutes.
3. Drizzle the cheese on top and cook for another two minutes or until the cheese has melted.
4. Serve with salad.

Nutrition

- Calories: 467
- Protein: 61g
- Fat: 22g

79. Air Fryer Pork Chop & Broccoli

Difficulty: Average
Preparation Time: 20 Minutes
Cooking Time: 20 Minutes
Servings: 2
Ingredients:

- 2 Cups Broccoli florets (1green)
- 2 Pieces Bone-in pork chop (1 lean)
- ½ Tsp. Paprika (1/4 condiment)
- 2 Tbsp. Avocado oil (1 healthy fat)
- ½ Tsp. Garlic powder (1/4 condiment)
- ½ Tsp. Onion powder (1/4 condiment)
- Two cloves of crushed garlic (1/4 condiment)
- 1 Teaspoon of Salt divided (1/4 condiment)

Directions:

1. Let the air fryer preheat to 350 degrees. Spray the basket with cooking oil
2. Add an oil spoon, onion powder, half a teaspoon. of salt, garlic powder, and paprika in a bowl mix well, rub this spice mixture on the sides of the pork chop
3. Add the pork chops to the fryer basket and cook for five minutes
4. Meanwhile, add an oil teaspoon, garlic, a half teaspoon of salt, and broccoli in a bowl and coat them well
5. Turn the pork chop and add the broccoli, let it cook for another five minutes.
6. Remove from the air fryer and serve.

Nutrition:

- Calories: 483
- Fat: 20g
- Protein: 23g

80. Mustard Glazed Air Fryer Pork Tenderloin

Difficulty: Average
Preparation Time: 10 Minutes
Cooking Time: 18 Minutes
Servings: 4
Ingredients:

- ¼ Cup Yellow mustard (½ green)
- One pork tenderloin (1 lean)
- ¼ Tsp. Salt (1/4 condiment)
- 3 Tbsp. Honey (½ healthy fat)
- 1/8 Tsp. Black pepper (1/4 condiment)
- 1 Tbsp. Minced garlic (1/4 condiment)
- 1 Tsp. Dried rosemary (1/4green)
- 1 Tsp. Italian seasoning (1/8 condiment)

Directions:

1. Using a knife, cut the top of the pork tenderloin. Add the garlic (minced) into the cuts. Then sprinkle with kosher salt and pepper.
2. In a bowl, add the honey, mustard, rosemary, and Italian seasoning mixture until well blended. Rub this mustard mix all over the pork.
3. Leave to marinate in the refrigerator for at least two hours.
4. Place the pork tenderloin in the basket of the air fryer. Cook for 18-20 minutes at 400°F. With an instant-read thermometer, verify that the internal temperature of the pig should be 145°F.
5. Remove from the air fryer and serve with a side of salad.

Nutrition:

- Calories: 390
- Protein: 59g
- Fat: 11g

81. Air Fryer Pork Taquitos

Difficulty: Average
Preparation Time: 10 Minutes
Cooking Time: 20 Minutes
Servings: 10
Ingredients:

- 3 Cups of Pork tenderloin, cooked & shredded (2 leans)
- 2 and ½ cups, fat-free Shredded mozzarella (1 healthy fat)
- 10 Small tortillas (1 healthy fat)
- Salsa for dipping (1 condiment)
- Juice of a lime (1/4 condiment)

Directions:

1. Allow the air fryer to preheat to 380°F.
2. Add the lime juice to the pork and mix well
3. With a damp towel over the tortilla, microwave for ten seconds to soften it
4. Add the pork filling and cheese on top in a tortilla, roll the tortilla tightly.
5. Situate the tortillas on a greased baking sheet
6. Sprinkle oil on the tortillas. Bake for 7-10 minutes or until the tortillas are golden; turn them halfway.
7. Serve with salad.

Nutrition:

- Calories: 253
- Fat: 18g
- Protein: 20g

82. Pork Rind Nachos

Difficulty: Average
Preparation Time: 5 Minutes
Cooking Time: 5 Minutes
Servings: 2
Ingredients:

- Tbsp. Of pork rinds (1 lean)
- 1/4 Cup shredded cooked chicken (½ lean)
- ½ Cup shredded Monterey jack cheese (1/4 healthy fat)
- 1/4 Cup sliced pickled jalapeños (1/4green)
- 1/4 Cup guacamole (1/4 healthy fat)
- 1/4 Cup full-fat sour cream (1/4 healthy fat)

Directions:

1. Place the pork rinds in a 6-inch round pan. Fill with grilled chicken and Monterey jack cheese. Place the pan in the basket with the air fryer.
2. Set the temperature to 370°F and set the timer for 5 minutes or until the cheese has melted.
3. Eat immediately with jalapeños, guacamole, and sour cream.

Nutrition:

- Calories: 295
- Protein: 30g
- Fat: 27g

83. Air Fried Jamaican Jerk Pork

Difficulty: Difficult
Preparation Time: 10 Minutes
Cooking Time: 20 Minutes
Servings: 4
Ingredients:

- Pork, cut into three-inch pieces (1 lean)
- ¼ Cup Jerk paste (1/4 condiment)

Directions:

1. Rub the jerk dough on all the pork pieces.
2. Chill to marinate for 4 hours in the refrigerator.
3. Allow the air fryer to preheat to 390°F. Spray with olive oil
4. Before placing it in the air fryer, allow the meat to rest for 20 minutes at room temperature.
5. Cook for 20 minutes at 390°F in the air fryer, turn halfway.
6. Remove from the air fryer and let sit for ten minutes before slicing.
7. Serve with microgreens.

Nutrition:

- Calories: 234
- Protein: 31g
- Fat: 9g

84. Beef Lunch Meatballs

Difficulty: Easy
Preparation Time: 10 Minutes
Cooking Time: 15 Minutes
Servings: 4
Ingredients:

- ½ Pound beef, ground (½ lean)
- ½ Pound Italian sausage, chopped (½ lean)
- ½ Tsp. Garlic powder (1/4 condiment)
- ½ Tsp. Onion powder (1/4 condiment)
- Salt and black pepper to the taste (1/4 condiment)
- ½ Cup cheddar cheese, grated (½ healthy fat)
- Mashed potatoes for serving (½ healthy fat)

Directions:

1. In a bowl, mix the beef with the sausage, garlic powder, onion powder, salt, pepper, and cheese, mix well and form 16 meatballs with this mixture.

2. Place the meatballs in your air fryer and cook them at 370°F for 15 minutes.

3. Serve the meatballs with some mashed potatoes on the side.

Nutrition:

- Calories: 132
- Fat: 6.7g
- Protein: 5.5g

85. Air Fryer Whole Wheat Crusted Pork Chops

Difficulty: Average
Preparation Time: 10 Minutes
Cooking Time: 12 Minutes
Servings: 4
Ingredients:

- 1 Cup whole-wheat breadcrumbs (½ healthy fat)
- ¼ Teaspoon salt (1/4 condiment)
- 2-4 Pieces pork chops (center cut and boneless) (2 leans)
- ½ Teaspoon Chili powder (1/4 condiment)
- 1 Tablespoon parmesan cheese (1/4 healthy fat)
- 1 ½ Teaspoons paprika (½ condiment)
- 1 Egg beaten (1 healthy fat)
- ½ Teaspoon Onion powder (1/4 condiment)
- ½ Teaspoon Granulated garlic (1/4 condiment)

Directions:

1. Allow the air fryer to preheat to 400°F.
2. Rub kosher salt on each side of the pork chops, let them rest
3. Add the beaten egg to a large bowl
4. Add the parmesan, breadcrumbs, garlic, pepper, paprika, chili powder, and onion powder to a bowl and mix well
5. Dip the pork chop in the egg and then in the breadcrumbs
6. Put it in the air fryer and spray it with oil.
7. Leave them to cook for 12 minutes at 400°F. Turn them upside down halfway through cooking. Cook for another six minutes.
8. Serve with salad.

Nutrition:

- Calories: 425
- Fat: 20g
- Protein: 31g

86. Air Fried Philly Cheesesteak Taquitos

Difficulty: Average
Preparation Time: 20 Minutes
Cooking Time: 6-8 Hours
Servings: 6
Ingredients:

- 1 Package Dry Italian dressing mix (1 condiment)
- 1 Pack Super Soft Corn Tortillas (1 healthy fat)
- 2 Pieces green peppers chopped (½ green)
- 12 Cups lean beef steak strips (3 leans)
- 2 Cups Beef stock (1 condiment)
- 1 Cup Lettuce shredded (½ green)
- 10 Slices provolone cheese (1 healthy fat)
- 1 Onion, chopped

Directions:

1. In a slow cooker, add onion, beef, stock, pepper, and seasonings.
2. Cover, then cook at low heat for 6 or 8 hours.
3. Heat the tortillas for two minutes in the microwave.
4. Allow the air fryer to preheat to 350°F.
5. Remove the cheesesteak from the slow cooker, add 2-3 tablespoons of steak to the tortilla.
6. Add some cheese, roll the tortilla well, and place in a deep fryer basket.
7. Make all the tortillas you want.
8. Lightly brush with olive oil
9. Cook for 6-8 minutes.
10. Flip the tortillas over and brush more oil as needed.
11. Serve with chopped lettuce and enjoy.

Nutrition:

- Calories: 220
- Protein: 21g
- Fat: 16g

Chapter 8. Snacks and Party Food

87. Salmon Sandwich With Avocado and Egg
Preparation Time: 15 Minutes
Cooking Time: 10 Minutes
Servings: 4
Ingredients:

- 8 Ounces (250g) smoked salmon, thinly sliced
- 1 Medium (200g) ripe avocado, thinly sliced
- 4 Large poached eggs (about 60g each)
- 4 Slices whole wheat bread (about 30g each)
- 2 Cups (60g) arugula or baby rocket
- Salt and freshly ground black pepper

Directions:

1. Place one bread slice on a plate top with arugula, avocado, salmon, and poached egg—season with salt and pepper. Repeat the procedure for the remaining ingredients.
2. Serve and enjoy.

Nutrition:

- Calories: 310
- Fat: 18.2g
- Carbohydrates: 16.4g
- Protein: 21.3g
- Sodium: 383mg

88. Tasty Onion and Cauliflower Dip

Preparation Time: 20 Minutes
Cooking Time: 30 Minutes
Servings: 24
Ingredients:

- 1 and ½ Cups chicken stock
- 1 Cauliflower head, florets separated
- ¼ Cup mayonnaise
- ½ Cup yellow onion, chopped
- ¾ Cup cream cheese
- ½ Teaspoon chili powder
- ½ Teaspoon cumin, ground
- ½ Teaspoon garlic powder
- Salt and black pepper to the taste

Directions:

1. Put the stock in a pot, add cauliflower and onion, heat up over medium heat, and cook for 30 minutes.
2. Add chili powder, salt, pepper, cumin, and garlic powder and stir.
3. Also, add cream cheese and stir a bit until it melts.
4. Blend using an immersion blender and mix with the mayo.
5. Transfer to a bowl and keep in the fridge for 2 hours before you serve it.
6. Enjoy!

Nutrition:

- Calories: 40 kcal
- Protein: 1.23g
- Fat: 3.31g
- Carbohydrates: 1.66g
- Sodium: 72mg

89. Marinated Eggs

Preparation Time: 2 Hours and 10 Minutes
Cooking Time: 7 Minutes
Servings: 4
Ingredients:

- 6 Eggs
- 1 and ¼ Cups of water
- ¼ Cup unsweetened rice vinegar
- 2 Tablespoons coconut aminos
- Salt and black pepper to the taste
- 2 Garlic cloves, minced
- 1 Teaspoon stevia
- 4 Ounces cream cheese
- 1 Tablespoon chives, chopped

Directions:

1. Put the eggs in a pot, add water to cover, bring to a boil over medium heat, cover and cook for 7 minutes.
2. Rinse eggs with cold water and leave them aside to cool down.
3. In a bowl, mix one cup of water with coconut aminos, vinegar, stevia, and garlic and whisk well.
4. Put the eggs in this mix, cover with a kitchen towel, and leave them aside for 2 hours, rotating from time to time.
5. Peel eggs, cut in halves, and put egg yolks in a bowl.
6. Add ¼ cup water, cream cheese, salt, pepper, and chives, and stir well.
7. Stuff egg whites with this mix and serve them.
8. Enjoy!

Nutrition:

- Calories: 289 kcal
- Protein: 15.86g
- Fat: 22.62g
- Carbohydrates: 4.52g
- Sodium: 288mg

90. Pumpkin Muffins

Preparation Time: 10 Minutes
Cooking Time: 15 Minutes
Servings: 18
Ingredients:

- ¼ Cup sunflower seed butter
- ¾ Cup pumpkin puree
- 2 Tablespoons flaxseed meal
- ¼ Cup coconut flour
- ½ Cup erythritol
- ½ Teaspoon nutmeg, ground
- 1 Teaspoon cinnamon, ground
- ½ Teaspoon baking soda
- 1 Egg
- ½ Teaspoon baking powder
- A pinch of salt

Directions:

1. In a bowl, mix butter with pumpkin puree and egg and blend well.
2. Add flaxseed meal, coconut flour, erythritol, baking soda, baking powder, nutmeg, cinnamon, and a pinch of salt and stir well.
3. Spoon this into a greased muffin pan, introduce in the oven at 350 degrees Fahrenheit and bake for 15 minutes.
4. Leave muffins to cool down and serve them as a snack.
5. Enjoy!

Nutrition:

- Calories: 65 kcal
- Protein: 2.82g
- Fat: 5.42g
- Carbohydrates: 2.27g
- Sodium: 57mg

91. Salmon Spinach and Cottage Cheese Sandwich

Preparation Time: 15 Minutes
Cooking Time: 10 Minutes
Servings: 4
Ingredients:

- 4 Ounces (125g) cottage cheese
- 1/4 Cup (15g) chives, chopped
- 1 Teaspoon (5g) capers
- ½ Teaspoon (2.5g) grated lemon rind
- 4 (2 oz. or 60g) Smoked salmon
- 2 Cups (60g) loose baby spinach
- 1 Medium (110g) red onion, sliced thinly
- 8 Slices rye bread (about 30g each)
- Kosher salt and freshly ground black pepper

Directions:

1. Preheat your griddle or Panini press.
2. Mix together cottage cheese, chives, capers, and lemon rind in a small bowl.
3. Spread and divide the cheese mixture on four bread slices. Top with spinach, onion slices, and smoked salmon.
4. Cover with remaining bread slices.
5. Grill the sandwiches until golden and grill marks form on both sides.
6. Transfer to a serving dish.
7. Serve and enjoy.

Nutrition:

- Calories: 261
- Fat: 9.9g
- Carbohydrates: 22.9g
- Protein: 19.9g
- Sodium: 1226mg

92. Sausage and Cheese Dip

Preparation Time: 10 Minutes
Cooking Time: 130 Minutes
Servings: 28
Ingredients:

- 8 Ounces cream cheese
- A pinch of salt and black pepper
- 16 Ounces sour cream
- 8 Ounces pepper jack cheese, chopped
- 15 Ounces canned tomatoes mixed with habaneros
- 1-pound Italian sausage, ground
- ¼ Cup green onions, chopped

Directions:

1. Heat up a pan over medium heat, add sausage, stir and cook until it browns.
2. Add tomatoes, mix, stir and cook for 4 minutes more.
3. Add a pinch of salt, pepper, and green onions, stir and cook for 4 minutes.
4. Spread the pepper jack cheese on the bottom of your slow cooker.
5. Add cream cheese, sausage mix, and sour cream, cover, and cook on High for 2 hours.
6. Uncover your slow cooker, stir dip, transfer to a bowl, and serve.
7. **Enjoy!**

Nutrition:

- Calories: 132 kcal
- Protein: 6.79g
- Fat: 9.58g
- Carbohydrates: 6.22g
- Sodium: 362mg

93. Pesto Crackers

Preparation Time: 10 Minutes
Cooking Time: 17 Minutes
Servings: 6
Ingredients:

- ½ Teaspoon baking powder
- Salt and black pepper to the taste
- 1 and ¼ Cups almond flour
- ¼ Teaspoon basil dried one garlic clove, minced
- 2 Tablespoons basil pesto
- A pinch of cayenne pepper
- 3 Tablespoons ghee

Directions:

1. In a bowl, mix salt, pepper, baking powder, and almond flour.
2. Add garlic, cayenne, and basil and stir.
3. Add pesto and whisk.
4. Also, add ghee and mix your dough with your finger.
5. Spread this dough on a lined baking sheet, introduce in the oven at 325 degrees F and bake for 17 minutes.
6. Leave aside to cool down, cut your crackers, and serve them as a snack.
7. Enjoy!

Nutrition:

- Calories: 9 kcal
- Protein: 0.41g
- Fat: 0.14g
- Carbohydrates: 1.86g
- Sodium: 2mg

94. Bacon Cheeseburger

Preparation Time: 10 Minutes
Cooking Time: 30 Minutes
Servings: 4
Ingredients:

- 1 lb. Lean ground beef
- 1/4 Cup chopped yellow onion
- 1 Clove garlic, minced
- 1 Tbsp. yellow mustard
- 1 Tbsp. Worcestershire sauce
- ½ Tsp. salt
- Cooking spray
- 4 Ultra-thin slices of cheddar cheese, cut into six equal-sized rectangular pieces
- 3 Pieces of turkey bacon, each cut into eight evenly-sized rectangular pieces
- 24 Dill pickle chips
- 4-6 Green leaf
- Lettuce leaves, torn into 24 small square-shaped pieces
- 12 Cherry tomatoes, sliced in half

Directions:

1. Pre-heat oven to 400°F.
2. Combine the garlic, salt, onion, Worcestershire sauce, and beef in a medium-sized bowl, and mix well.
3. Form the mixture into 24 small meatballs.
4. Put meatballs onto a foil-lined baking sheet and cook for 12-15 minutes.
5. Leave the oven on.
6. Top every meatball with a piece of cheese, then go back to the oven until cheese melts for about 2 to 3 minutes.
7. Let the meatballs cool.
8. To assemble bites, on a toothpick, put a cheese-covered meatball, a piece of bacon, a piece of lettuce, pickle chip, and a tomato half.

Nutrition:

- Fat: 14g
- Cholesterol: 41mg
- Carbohydrates: 30g
- Protein: 15g

95. Cheeseburger Pie

Preparation Time: 20 Minutes
Cooking Time: 90 Minutes
Servings: 4
Ingredients:

- 1 Large spaghetti squash
- 1 lb. Lean ground beef
- 1/4 Cup diced onion
- 2 Eggs
- 1/3 Cup low-fat, plain Greek yogurt
- 2 Tablespoons tomato sauce
- ½ Tsp. Worcestershire sauce
- 2/3 Cups reduced-fat, shredded cheddar cheese
- 2 oz. Dill pickle slices
- Cooking spray

Directions:

1. Preheat oven to 400°F. Slice spaghetti squash in half lengthwise; dismiss pulp and seeds.
2. Spray insides with cooking spray.
3. Place squash halves cut-side-down onto a foil-lined baking sheet, and bake for 30 minutes.
4. Once cooked, let it cool before scraping squash flesh with a fork to remove spaghetti-like strands; set aside.
5. Push squash strands in the bottom and up sides of the greased pie pan, creating an even layer.
6. Meanwhile, set up pie filling.
7. In a lightly greased, medium-sized skillet, cook beef and onion over medium heat for 8 to 10 minutes, sometimes stirring, until meat is brown.
8. Drain and remove from heat.
9. In a medium-sized bowl, whisk together eggs, tomato sauce, Greek yogurt, and Worcestershire sauce. Stir in ground beef mixture.
10. Pour pie filling over the squash crust.
11. Sprinkle meat filling with cheese, and then top with dill pickle slices.
12. Bake for 40 minutes.

Nutrition:

- Calories: 409 Cal
- Fat: 24.49g
- Carbohydrates: 15.06g
- Protein: 30.69g

96. Smoked Salmon and Cheese on Rye Bread

Preparation Time: 15 Minutes
Cooking Time: 10 Minutes
Servings: 4
Ingredients:

- 8 Ounces (250g) smoked salmon, thinly sliced
- 1/3 Cup (85g) mayonnaise
- 2 Tablespoons (30ml) lemon juice
- 1 Tablespoon (15g) Dijon mustard
- 1 Teaspoon (3g) garlic, minced
- 4 Slices cheddar cheese (about 2 oz. or 30g each)
- 8 Slices rye bread (about 2 oz. or 30g each)
- 8 (15g) Romaine lettuce leaves
- Salt and freshly ground black pepper

Directions:

1. Mix together the mayonnaise, lemon juice, mustard, and garlic in a small bowl. Flavor with salt and pepper and set aside.
2. Spread dressing on four bread slices. Top with lettuce, salmon, and cheese. Cover with remaining rye bread slices.
3. Serve and enjoy.

Nutrition:

- Calories: 365
- Fat: 16.6g
- Carbohydrates: 31.6g
- Protein: 18.8g
- Sodium: 951mg

97. Chicken and Mushrooms

Preparation Time: 10 Minutes
Cooking Time: 15 Minutes
Servings: 6
Ingredients:

- 2 Chicken breasts
- 1 Cup of sliced white champignons
- 1 Cup of sliced green chilies
- ½ Cup scallions hacked
- 1 Teaspoon of chopped garlic
  1 Cup of low-fat cheddar shredded cheese (1-1,5 lb. grams fat
- / ounce)
- 1 Tablespoon of olive oil
- 1 Tablespoon of butter

Directions:

1. Fry the chicken breasts with olive oil.
2. When needed, add salt and pepper.
3. Grill the chicken breasts on a plate with a grill.
4. For every serving, weigh 4 ounces of chicken. (Make two servings, save leftovers for another meal).
5. In a buttered pan, stir in mushrooms, green peppers, scallions, and garlic until smooth and a little dark.
6. Place the chicken on a baking platter.
7. Cover with the mushroom combination.
8. Top on ham.
9. Place the cheese in a 350 oven until it melts.

Nutrition:

- Carbohydrates: 2g
- Protein: 23g
- Fat: 11g
- Cholesterol: 112mg
- Sodium: 198mg
- Potassium: 261mg

98. Chicken Enchilada Bake

Preparation Time: 20 Minutes
Cooking Time: 50 Minutes
Servings: 5
Ingredients:

- 5 oz. Shredded chicken breast (boil and shred ahead) or 99 percent fat-free white chicken can be used in a pan.
- 1 Can tomato paste
- 1 Low sodium chicken broth can be fat-free
- 1/4 Cup cheese with low-fat mozzarella
- 1 Tablespoon oil
- 1 Tbsp. of salt
  Ground cumin, chili powder, garlic powder, oregano, and
- onion powder (all to taste)
- 1 to 2 Zucchinis sliced longways (similar to lasagna noodles)
- into thin lines Sliced (optional) olives

Directions:

1. Add olive oil in a saucepan over medium/high heat, stir in tomato paste and seasonings, and heat in chicken broth for 2-3 min.
2. Stirring regularly to boil, turn heat to low for 15 min.
3. Set aside and cool to ambient temperature.
4. Dredge a zucchini strip through enchilada sauce and lay flat on the pan's bottom in a small baking pan.
5. Next, add the chicken a little less than 1/4 cup of enchilada sauce and mix it.
6. Attach the chicken to cover and end the baking tray.
7. Sprinkle some bacon over the chicken.

8. Add another layer of the soaked enchilada sauce zucchini (similar to lasagna making).
9. When needed, cover with the remaining cheese and olives on top—bake for 35 to 40 minutes.
10. Keep an eye on them.
11. When the cheese starts getting golden, cover with foil.
12. Serve and enjoy!

Nutrition:

- Calories: 312 Cal
- Carbohydrates: 21.3g
- Protein: 27g
- Fat: 10.2g

99. Salmon Feta and Pesto Wrap

Preparation Time: 15 Minutes
Cooking Time: 10 Minutes
Servings: 4
Ingredients:

- 8 Ounces (250g) smoked salmon fillet, thinly sliced
- 1 Cup (150g) feta cheese
- 8 (15g) Romaine lettuce leaves
- 4 (6-inch) Pita bread
- 1/4 Cup (60g) basil pesto sauce

Directions:

1. Place one pita bread on a plate. Top with lettuce, salmon, feta cheese, and pesto sauce. Fold or roll to enclose filling. Repeat the procedure for the remaining ingredients.
2. Serve and enjoy.

Nutrition:

- Calories: 379
- Fat: 17.7g
- Carbohydrates: 36.6g
- Protein: 18.4g
- Sodium: 554mg

100. Pan-Fried Trout

Preparation Time: 15 Minutes
Cooking Time: 10 Minutes
Servings: 4
Ingredients:

- 1 ¼ Pounds trout fillets
- 1/3 Cup white, or yellow, cornmeal
- ¼ Teaspoon anise seeds
- ¼ Teaspoon black pepper
- ½ Cup minced cilantro, or parsley
- Vegetable cooking spray
- Lemon wedges

Directions:

1. Coat the fish with combined cornmeal, spices, and cilantro, pressing them gently into the fish. Spray a large skillet with cooking spray; heat over medium heat until hot.
2. Add fish and cook until it is tender and flakes with a fork, about 5 minutes on each side. Serve with lemon wedges.

Nutrition:

- Calories: 207
- Total Carbohydrates: 19g
- Cholesterol: 27mg
- Total Fat: 16g
- Fiber: 4g
- Protein: 18g

101. Glazed Bananas in Phyllo Nut Cups

Preparation Time: 30 Minutes
Cooking Time: 45 Minutes
Servings: 6 Servings
Ingredients:

- 3/4 Cups shelled pistachios
- ½ Cup sugar
- 1 Teaspoon. ground cinnamon
- 4 Sheets phyllo dough (14 inches x 9 inches)
- 1/4 Cup butter, melted

Sauce:

- 3/4 Cup butter, cubed
- 3/4 Cup packed brown sugar
- 3 Medium-firm bananas, sliced
- 1/4 Teaspoon. ground cinnamon
- 3 to 4 Cups vanilla ice cream

Directions:

1. Finely chop sugar and pistachios in a food processor; move to a bowl, then mix in cinnamon. Slice each phyllo sheet into six four-inch squares, get rid of the trimmings. Pile the squares, then use plastic wrap to cover.
2. Slather melted butter on each square one at a time, then scatter a heaping tablespoonful of pistachio mixture. Pile three squares, flip each at an angle to misalign the corners. Force each stack on the sides and bottom of an oiled eight ounces custard cup. Bake for 15-20 minutes in a 350 degrees F oven until golden; cool for 5 minutes. Move to a wire rack to cool completely.
3. Melt and boil brown sugar and butter in a saucepan to make the sauce; lower heat. Mix in cinnamon and bananas gently; heat completely. Put ice cream in the phyllo cups until full, then put banana sauce on top. Serve right away.

Nutrition:

- Calories: 735
- Total Carbohydrate: 82g
- Cholesterol: 111mg
- Total Fat: 45g
- Fiber: 3g
- Protein: 7g
- Sodium: 468mg

102. Salmon Cream Cheese and Onion on Bagel

Preparation Time: 15 Minutes
Cooking Time: 10 Minutes
Servings: 4
Ingredients:

- 8 Ounces (250g) smoked salmon fillet, thinly sliced
- ½ Cup (125g) cream cheese
- 1 Medium (110g) onion, thinly sliced
- 4 Bagels (about 80g each), split
- 2 Tablespoons (7g) fresh parsley, chopped
- Freshly ground black pepper, to taste

Directions:

4. Spread the cream cheese on each bottom's half of bagels. Top with salmon and onion, season with pepper, sprinkle with parsley and then cover with bagel tops.
5. Serve and enjoy.

Nutrition:

- Calories: 309
- Fat: 14.1g
- Carbohydrates: 32.0g
- Protein: 14.7g
- Sodium: 571mg

219. Salmon Apple Salad Sandwich

Preparation Time: 15 Minutes
Cooking Time: 10 Minutes
Servings: 4
Ingredients:

- 4 Ounces (125g) canned pink salmon, drained and flaked
- 1 Medium (180g) red apple, cored and diced
- 1 Celery stalk (about 60g), chopped
- 1 Shallot (about 40g), finely chopped
- 1/3 Cup (85g) light mayonnaise
- 8 Whole grain bread slices (about 30g each), toasted
- 8 (15g) Romaine lettuce leaves
- Salt and freshly ground black pepper

Directions:

1. Combine the salmon, apple, celery, shallot, and mayonnaise in a mixing bowl—season with salt and pepper.
2. Place one bread slice on a plate, top with lettuce and salmon salad, and then cover it with another slice of bread—repeat the procedure for the remaining ingredients.
3. Serve and enjoy.

Nutrition:

- Calories: 315
- Fat: 11.3g
- Carbohydrates: 40.4g
- Protein: 15.1g
- Sodium: 469mg

103. Greek Baklava

Preparation Time: 20 Minutes
Cooking Time: 20 Minutes
Servings: 18
Ingredients:

- 1 (16 oz.) Package phyllo dough
- 1 lb. Chopped nuts
- 1 Cup butter
- 1 Teaspoon ground cinnamon
- 1 Cup water
- 1 Cup white sugar
- 1 Teaspoon vanilla extract
- ½ Cup honey

Directions:

1. Preheat the oven to 175°C or 350°Fahrenheit. Spread butter on the sides and bottom of a 9- by 13-inch pan.
2. Chop the nuts, then mix with cinnamon; set it aside. Unfurl the phyllo dough, then halve the whole stack to fit the pan. Use a damp cloth to cover the phyllo to prevent drying as you proceed. Put two phyllo sheets in the pan, then butter well. Repeat to make eight layered phyllo sheets. Scatter 2-3 tablespoons of the nut mixture over the sheets, then place two more phyllo sheets on top, butter, sprinkle with nuts—layer as you go. The final layer should be six to eight phyllo sheets deep.
3. Make square or diamond shapes with a sharp knife up to the bottom of the pan. You can slice into four long rows for diagonal shapes. Bake until crisp and golden for 50 minutes.
4. Meanwhile, boil water and sugar until the sugar melts to make the sauce; mix in honey and vanilla. Let it simmer for 20 minutes.
5. Take the baklava out of the oven, then drizzle with sauce right away; cool. Serve the baklava in cupcake papers. You can also freeze them without cover. The baklava will turn soggy when wrapped.

Nutrition:

- Calories: 393
- Total Carbohydrate: 37.5g
- Cholesterol: 27mg
- Total Fat: 25.9g
- Protein: 6.1g
- Sodium: 196mg

104. Easy Salmon Burger

Preparation Time: 15 minutes
Cooking Time: 15 minutes
Servings: 6
Ingredients:

- 16 Ounces (450g) pink salmon, minced
- 1 Cup (250g) prepared mashed potatoes
- 1 Medium (110g) onion, chopped
- 1 Stalk celery (about 60g), finely chopped
- 1 Large egg (about 60g), lightly beaten
- 2 Tablespoons (7g) fresh cilantro, chopped
- 1 Cup (100g) breadcrumbs
- Vegetable oil, for deep frying
- Salt and freshly ground black pepper

Directions:

1. Combine the salmon, mashed potatoes, onion, celery, egg, and cilantro in a mixing bowl. Season to taste and mix thoroughly. Spoon about 2 Tablespoons of the mixture, roll in breadcrumbs, and then form into small patties.
2. Heat oil in a non-stick frying pan. Cook your salmon patties for 5 minutes on each side or until golden brown and crispy.
3. Serve in burger buns and with coleslaw on the side if desired.
4. Enjoy.

Nutrition:

- Calories: 230
- Fat: 7.9g
- Carbs: 20.9g
- Protein: 18.9g
- Sodium: 298mg

105. White Bean Dip

Preparation Time: 10 Minutes
Cooking Time: 0 Minutes
Servings: 4
Ingredients:

- 15 Ounces canned white beans, drained and rinsed
- 6 Ounces canned artichoke hearts, drained and quartered
- 4 Garlic cloves, minced
- 1 Tablespoon basil, chopped
- 2 Tablespoons olive oil
- Juice of ½ lemon
- Zest of ½ lemon, grated
- Salt and black pepper to the taste

Directions:

1. In your food processor, combine the beans with the artichokes and the rest of the ingredients except the oil and pulse well.
2. Add the oil gradually, pulse the mix again, divide into cups and serve as a party dip.

Nutrition:

- Calories: 274
- Fat: 11.7g
- Fiber: 6.5g
- Carbs: 18.5g
- Protein: 16.5g

106. Grilled Salmon Burger

Preparation Time: 15 Minutes
Cooking Time: 10 Minutes
Servings: 4
Ingredients:

- 16 Ounces (450g) pink salmon fillet, minced
- 1 Cup (250g) prepared mashed potatoes
- 1 Shallot (about 40g), chopped
- 1 Large egg (about 60g), lightly beaten
- 2 Tablespoons (7g) fresh coriander, chopped
- 4 Hamburger buns (about 60g each), split
- 1 Large tomato (about 150g), sliced
- 8 (15g) Romaine lettuce leaves
- 1/4 Cup (60g) mayonnaise
- Salt and freshly ground black pepper
- Cooking oil spray

Directions:

1. Combine the salmon, mashed potatoes, shallot, egg, and coriander in a mixing bowl—season with salt and pepper.
2. Spoon about two tablespoons of mixture and form into patties.
3. Preheat your grill or griddle on high—grease with cooking oil spray.
4. Grill the salmon patties for 4-5 minutes on each side or until cooked through. Transfer to a clean plate and cover to keep warm.
5. Spread some mayonnaise on the bottom half of the buns. Top with lettuce, salmon patty, and tomato. Cover with bun tops.
6. Serve and enjoy.

Nutrition:

- Calories: 395
- Fat: 18.0g
- Carbohydrates: 38.8g
- Protein: 21.8g
- Sodium: 383mg

Chapter 9. Desserts Recipes

107. Chocolate Bars
Preparation Time: 10 Minutes
Cooking Time: 20 Minutes
Servings: 16
Ingredients:

- 15 oz. Cream cheese softened
- 15 oz. Unsweetened dark chocolate
- 1 Tsp. Vanilla
- 10 Drops liquid stevia

Directions:

1. Grease an 8-inch square dish and set it aside.
2. In a saucepan, dissolve chocolate over low heat.
3. Add stevia and vanilla and stir well.
4. Remove the pan from heat and set it aside.
5. Add cream cheese into the blender and blend until smooth.
6. Add the melted chocolate mixture into the cream cheese and blend until just combined.
7. Transfer mixture into the prepared dish and spread evenly, and place in the refrigerator until firm.
8. Slice and serve.

Nutrition:

- Calories: 230
- Fat: 24g
- Carbs: 7.5g
- Sugar: 0.1g
- Protein: 6g
- Cholesterol: 29mg

108. Blueberry Muffins

Preparation Time: 15 Minutes
Cooking Time: 35 Minutes
Servings: 12
Ingredients:

- 2 Eggs
- ½ Cup fresh blueberries
- 1 Cup heavy cream
- 2 Cups almond flour
- 1/4 Tsp. lemon zest
- ½ Tsp. lemon extract
- 1 Tsp. baking powder
- 5 Drops stevia
- 1/4 Cup butter, melted

Directions:

1. Heat the cooker to 350°F. Line muffin tin with cupcake liners and set aside.
2. Add eggs into the bowl and whisk until mix.
3. Add remaining ingredients and mix to combine.
4. Pour mixture into the prepared muffin tin and bake for 25 minutes.
5. Serve and enjoy.

Nutrition:

- Calories: 190
- Fat: 17g
- Carbs: 5g
- Sugar: 1g
- Protein: 5g
- Cholesterol: 55mg

109. Chocolate Fondue

Preparation Time: 5 Minutes
Cooking Time: 10 Minutes
Servings: 2
Ingredients:

- 1 Cup water
- ½ Tsp. sugar
- ½ Cup coconut cream
- ¾ Cup dark chocolate, chopped

Directions:

1. Pour the water into your Instant Pot.
2. To a heatproof bowl, add the chocolate, sugar, and coconut cream.
3. Place in the Instant Pot.
4. Seal the lid, select MANUAL, and cook for 2 minutes. When ready, do a quick release and carefully open the lid. Stir well and serve immediately.

Nutrition:

- Calories: 216
- Fat: 17g
- Carbs: 11g
- Protein: 2g

110. Apple Crisp

Preparation Time: 10 Minutes
Cooking Time: 13 Minutes
Servings: 2
Ingredients:

- 2 Apples, sliced into chunks
- 1 Tsp. Cinnamon
- ¼ Cup rolled oats
- 1/4 Cup brown sugar
- ½ Cup of water

Directions:

1. Put all the listed ingredients in the pot and mix well.
2. Seal the pot, choose MANUAL mode, and cook at HIGH pressure for 8 minutes.
3. Release the pressure naturally and let sit for 5 minutes or until the sauce has thickened.
4. Serve and enjoy.

Nutrition:

- Calories: 218
- Fat: 5mg
- Carbs: 54g

111. Yogurt Mint

Preparation Time: 5 Minutes
Cooking Time: 10 Minutes
Servings: 2
Ingredients:

- 1 Cup of water
- 5 Cups of milk
- ¾ Cup plain yogurt
- ¼ Cup fresh mint
- 1 Tbsp. maple syrup

Directions:

1. Add one water cup to the Instant Pot Pressure Cooker.
2. Press the STEAM function button and adjust it to 1 minute.
3. Once done, add the milk, then press the YOGURT function button and allow boiling.
4. Add yogurt and fresh mint, then stir well.
5. Pour into a glass and add maple syrup.
6. Enjoy.

Nutrition:

- Calories: 25
- Fat: 0.5g
- Carbs: 5g
- Protein: 2g

112. Raspberry Compote

Preparation Time: 11 Minutes
Cooking Time: 30 Minutes
Servings: 2
Ingredients:

- 1 Cup raspberries
- ½ Cup Swerve
- 1 Tsp. freshly grated lemon zest
- 1 Tsp. vanilla extract
- 2 Cups water

Directions:

1. Press the SAUTÉ button on your Instant Pot, then add all the listed ingredients.
2. Stir well and pour in one cup of water.
3. Cook for 5 minutes, continually stirring, then pour in 1 more cup of water and press the CANCEL button.
4. Secure the lid properly, press the MANUAL button, and set the timer to 15 minutes on LOW pressure.
5. When the timer buzzes, press the CANCEL button and release the pressure naturally for 10minutes.
6. Move the pressure handle to the "venting" position to release any remaining pressure and open the lid.
7. Let it cool before serving.

Nutrition:

- Calories: 48
- Fat: 0.5g
- Carbs: 5g
- Protein: 1g

113. Braised Apples

Preparation Time: 5 Minutes
Cooking Time: 12 Minutes
Servings: 2
Ingredients:

- 2 Cored apples
- ½ Cup of water
- ½ Cup red wine
- 3 Tbsp. sugar
- ½ Tsp. ground cinnamon

Directions:

1. In the bottom of the Instant Pot, add the water and place the apples.
2. Pour wine on top and sprinkle with sugar and cinnamon. Close the lid carefully and cook for 10 minutes at HIGH PRESSURE.
3. When done, do a quick pressure release.
4. Transfer the apples onto serving plates and top with cooking liquid.
5. Serve immediately.

Nutrition:

- Calories: 245
- Fat: 0.5g
- Carbs: 53g
- Protein: 1g

114. Rice Pudding

Preparation Time: 5 Minutes
Cooking Time: 12 Minutes
Servings: 2
Ingredients:

- ½ Cup short grain rice
- ¼ Cup of sugar
- 1 Cinnamon stick
- 1½ Cup milk
- 1 Slice lemon peel
- Salt to taste

Directions:

1. Rinse the rice under cold water.
2. Put the rice, milk, cinnamon stick, sugar, salt, and lemon peel inside the Instant Pot Pressure Cooker.
3. Close the lid, lock it in place, and make sure to seal the valve. Press the PRESSURE button and cook for 10 minutes on HIGH.
4. When the timer beeps, choose the QUICK PRESSURE release. This will take about 2 minutes.
5. Remove the lid. Open the pressure cooker and discard the lemon peel and cinnamon stick. Spoon in a serving bowl and serve.

Nutrition:

- Calories: 111
- Fat: 6g
- Carbs: 21g
- Protein: 3g

115. Rhubarb Dessert

Preparation Time: 4 Minutes
Cooking Time: 5 Minutes
Servings: 2
Ingredients:

- 3 Cups rhubarb, chopped
- 1 Tbsp. ghee, melted
- 1/3 Cup water
- 1 Tbsp. stevia
- 1 Tsp. vanilla extract

Directions:

1. Put all the listed ingredients in your Instant Pot, cover, and cook on HIGH for 5 minutes.
2. Divide into small bowls and serve cold.
3. Enjoy!

Nutrition:

- Calories: 83
- Fat: 2g
- Carbs: 2g
- Protein: 2g

116. Wine Figs

Preparation Time: 5 Minutes
Cooking Time: 3 Minutes
Servings: 2
Ingredients:

- ½ Cup pine nuts
- 1 Cup red wine
- 1 lb. Figs
- Sugar, as needed

Directions:

1. Slowly pour the wine and sugar into the Instant Pot.
2. Arrange the trivet inside it; place the figs over it. Close the lid and lock. Ensure that you have sealed the valve to avoid leakage.
3. Press MANUAL mode and set the timer to 3 minutes.
4. After the timer reads zero, you have to press CANCEL and quick-release pressure.
5. Carefully remove the lid.
6. Divide figs into bowls, and drizzle wine from the pot over them.
7. Top with pine nuts and enjoy.

Nutrition:

- Calories: 95
- Fat: 3g
- Carbs: 5g
- Protein: 2g

117. Chia Pudding

Preparation Time: 20 Minutes
Cooking Time: 0 Minutes
Servings: 2
Ingredients:

- 4 Tbsp. chia seeds
- 1 Cup unsweetened coconut milk
- ½ Cup raspberries

Directions:

1. Add raspberry and coconut milk into a blender and blend until smooth.
2. Pour mixture into a glass jar.
3. Add chia seeds in a jar and stir well.
4. Seal the jar with a lid and shake well and place in the refrigerator for 3 hours.
5. Serve chilled and enjoy.

Nutrition:

- Calories: 360
- Fat: 33g
- Carbs: 13g
- Sugar: 5g
- Protein: 6g
  Cholesterol: 0mg

Chapter 10. Air Fryer Meals and Breakfast Recipes

118. Cloud Focaccia Bread Breakfast

Difficulty: Difficult
Preparation Time: 10 Minutes
Cooking Time: 30 Minutes
Servings: 2
Ingredients:

- 2 Medium eggs, separate yolk, and white (1 healthy fat)
- 1½ Tbsp. Cream cheese, low fat (1 healthy fat)
- ½ Package sweetener, no-calorie (½ condiment)
- ¼ Tsp. Tartar cream (1/4 condiment)

For Focaccia Bread:

- ½ Tsp. Olive oil
- ½ Tsp. Rosemary (½ green)
- 1/8 Tsp. Salt (1/4 condiment)

Directions:

1. Combine thoroughly cream cheese, egg yolks, and the sweetener in a medium bowl.
2. Beat the egg whites in a large bowl along with tartar cream until the whites become stiff peaks.
3. Now carefully fold the yolk mixture into the egg whites without breaking the whites.
4. Line a parchment paper in the air fryer baking tray and place four scoops of the mixture without overlapping one another.
5. Set the temperature to 150°C and bake for 20 minutes.
6. Take out the bread, brush olive oil on top and sprinkle Rosemary and salt.
7. Place it again into the air fryer and bake for further 10 minutes until the top becomes golden brown.
8. After baking, allow it to cool down before serving.

Nutrition:

- Calories: 90
- Fat: 6.5g
- Protein: 6g

119. Cloud Garlic Bread Breakfast

Difficulty: Difficult
Preparation Time: 10 Minutes
Cooking Time: 30 Minutes
Servings: 2
Ingredients:

- 2 Eggs, medium (separate yolk and white) (1 healthy fat)
- 1½ Tbsp. Cream cheese, low fat (1 healthy fat)
- ½ Packet Sweetener, no-calorie (½ condiment)
- ¼ Tsp. Tartar cream (1/4 condiment)

For Garlic Bread:

- 1 Tsp. Butter, unsalted, melted (½ healthy fat)
- 1/8 Tsp. Garlic powder (1/4 condiment)
- ¼ Tsp. Italian seasoning (1/4 condiment)
- 1/8 Tsp. Salt (1/4 condiment)

Directions:

1. Combine thoroughly cream cheese, egg yolks, and the sweetener in a medium bowl.
2. Beat the egg whites in a large bowl along with tartar cream until the whites become stiff peaks.
3. Now carefully fold the yolk mixture into the egg whites without breaking the whites.
4. Line a parchment paper in the air fryer baking tray and place four scoops of the mixture without overlapping one another.
5. Set the temperature to 150°C and bake for 20 minutes.
6. Take out the bread, and brush butter on top and sprinkle the seasoning, garlic powder, and salt.
7. Place it again into the air fryer and bake for further 10 minutes until the top becomes golden brown.
8. After baking, allow it to cool before serving.

Nutrition:

- Calories: 115
- Fat: 8.8g
- Protein: 6g

120. Cheesy Broccoli Bites

Difficulty: Average
Preparation Time: 5 Minutes
Cooking Time: 40 Minutes
Servings: 2
Ingredients:

- 3 Cups Frozen broccoli (2greens)
- ¼ Cup Scallions, thinly sliced (½ green)
- 2 Eggs (1 healthy fat)
- 1 Cup Cottage cheese (½ healthy fat)
- ¾ Cup Mozzarella cheese, grated (½ healthy fat)
- ¼ Cup Parmesan cheese, shredded (1/4 healthy fat)
- 1 Tsp. Olive oil (½ condiment)
- ½ Tsp. Garlic powder (½ condiment)
- 1/8 Tsp. Salt (1/4 condiment)
- 2 Cups Water (1 healthy fat)

Directions:

1. Preheat the air fryer to 190°C.
2. Place the broccoli in an air fryer, save bowl, and pour water.
3. Air fryer it for 10 minutes until the broccoli becomes tender.
4. Drain the water and transfer the broccoli into the blender.
5. Blitz it until it chopped well.
6. Now add cottage cheese, scallions, parmesan, mozzarella, eggs, olive oil, salt, and garlic into the blender.
7. Pulse it until it gets mixed well.
8. Transfer it to 12 muffin tins evenly after greasing them.
9. Place it in the air fryer and bake for 30 minutes until the filling becomes firm and its top turns to a golden brown.
10. After baking, remove them from the air fryer.
11. Allow it to settle down the heat and serve.

Nutrition:

- Calories: 366
- Fat: 15.1g
- Protein: 41g

121. Portabella Mushrooms Stuffed With Cheese

Difficulty: Difficult
Preparation Time: 15 Minutes
Cooking Time: 17 Minutes
Servings: 2
Ingredients:

- 4 Portabella mushroom caps, large (2 leans)
- 1 Tbsp. Soy sauce (½ condiment)
- 1 Tbsp. Lemon juice (½ condiment)
- 1 Tsp. Olive oil, divided (1/4 condiment)
- 2 Cups Mozzarella cheese, low fat, grated (1 healthy fat)
- ½ Cup Tomato, fresh, diced (½ green)
- 1 Garlic Clove, finely grated (1/4green)
- 1 Tbsp. Cilantro, fresh, chopped (1/4green)

Directions:

1. Make bowls by scooping the flesh from the interior of the mushroom caps.
2. Set the air fryer temperature to 200°C and preheat.
3. Mix the soy sauce, lemon juice, and half a portion of olive oil in a small bowl.
4. Marinate the mixture on the mushroom cap both inside and outside.
5. Line foil-coated baking paper in the air fryer tray.
6. Place the marinated mushroom cap in the tray and bake for 10 minutes until they become tender.
7. Now combine tomatoes, mozzarella, garlic, remaining olive oil, and Italian seasoning in a medium bowl.
8. Fill the mushroom caps with the mixture evenly.
9. Bake it in the air fryer for 7 minutes until the cheese starts to melt.
10. Sprinkle cilantro on top and serve.

Nutrition:

- Calories: 250
- Fat: 4.4g
- Protein: 40g

122. Bell-Pepper Wrapped in Tortilla

Difficulty: Easy
Preparation Time: 5 Minutes
Cooking Time: 15 Minutes
Servings: 1
Ingredients:

- 1/4 Small red bell pepper (½ greens)
- 1/4 Tablespoon water (½ condiment)
- 1 Large tortilla (1 healthy fat)
- 1-piece Commercial vegan nuggets, chopped (3 leans)
- Mixed greens for garnish (6greens)

Directions:

1. Preheat the Instant Crisp Air Fryer to 400°F.
2. In a skillet heated over medium heat, water sautés the vegan nuggets and bell pepper. Set aside.
3. Place filling inside the corn tortilla.
4. Fold the tortilla, place them inside the Instant Crisp Air Fryer, and cook for 15 minutes until the tortilla wrap is crispy.
5. Serve with mixed greens on top.

Nutrition:

- Calories: 548
- Fat: 21g
- Protein: 46g

123. Air Fried Cauliflower Ranch Chips

Difficulty: Easy
Preparation Time: 5 Minutes
Cooking Time: 12 Minutes
Servings: 2
Ingredients:

- ½ Cup Raw cauliflower, grated (1/4green)
- ¼ Tsp. Parsley (1/8green)
- ¼ Tsp. Basil (1/8green)
- ¼ Tsp. Dill (1/8green)
- ¼ Tsp. Chives (1/8green)
- ¼ Tsp. Garlic powder (1/8 condiment)
- ¼ Tsp. Onion powder (1/8 condiment)
- ¼ Tsp. Pepper, ground (1/8 condiment)
- ¼ Cup Parmesan cheese (1/8 healthy fat)
- Cooking spray as required (½ healthy fat)

Directions:

1. Preheat the air fryer to 230°C.

2. Using a medium bowl, mix all the ingredients.
3. Line the air fryer baking tray with parchment paper.
4. Scoop one tablespoon of mixture and place it on the parchment paper without overlapping one another.
5. Bake for 12 minutes by flipping side halfway through.
6. Serve hot.

Nutrition:

- Calories: 65
- Fat: 3.6g
- Protein: 4g

124. Brine & Spinach Egg Air Fried Muffins

Difficulty: Difficult
Preparation Time: 10 Minutes
Cooking Time: 25 Minutes
Servings: 2
Ingredients:
For the Egg Muffin:

- 4 Eggs (2 healthy fat)
- 1 Cup Liquid egg whites (½ healthy fat)
- ¼ Cup Greek yogurt, plain, low fat (½ healthy fat)
- ¼ Tsp. Salt (1/4 condiment)

For Brie, Spinach & Mushroom Mix:

- 1 oz. Brie (½ green)
- 5 oz. Spinach, frozen, coarsely chopped (2greens)
- 1 Cup Mushrooms, chopped (½ green)

Directions:

1. Thaw the frozen spinach for 10 minutes.
2. Wash all the vegetables separately and pat dry.
3. Preheat the air fryer to 190°C.
4. In a large bowl, combine Greek yogurt, egg whites, eggs, cheese, and salt.
5. Add all the vegetables to the bowl, mix, and combine well.
6. Take 12 muffin tins and lightly spray with cooking oil.
7. Transfer the mixture evenly into the muffin tins.
8. Place them in the air fryer and bake for 25 minutes until the center portion becomes hard.
9. Do a toothpick test by inserting it in the center and check if it comes out clean.
10. Take it out from the air fryer and allow it to settle down the heat before serving.
11. Enjoy your muffin.

Nutrition:

- Calories: 278
- Fat: 13.1g
- Protein: 33g

125. Coconut Battered Cauliflower Bites

Difficulty: Average
Preparation Time: 5 Minutes
Cooking Time: 20 Minutes
Servings: 1
Ingredients:

- Salt and pepper to taste (2 condiments)
- 1 Flax egg or one tablespoon flaxseed meal + 3 tablespoon water (1 healthy fat)
- 1 Small cauliflower, cut into florets (2greens)
- 1 Teaspoon mixed spice (1 condiment)
- ½ Teaspoon mustard powder (1 condiment)
- 2 Tablespoons maple syrup (2 healthy fats)
- 1 Clove of garlic, minced (1green)
- 2 Tablespoons soy sauce (2 condiments)
- 1/3 Cup oats flour (½ healthy fat)
- 1/3 Cup plain flour (½ healthy fat)
- 1/3 Cup desiccated coconut (½ lean)

Directions:

1. In a mixing bowl, mix oats, flour, and desiccated coconut. Season with salt and pepper to taste. Set aside.
2. In another bowl, place the flax egg and add a pinch of salt to taste. Set aside.
3. Season the cauliflower with mixed spice and mustard powder.
4. Dredge the florets in the flax egg first, then in the flour mixture.
5. Place inside the Instant Crisp Air Fryer, lock the air fryer lid, and cook at 400°F or 15 minutes.
6. Meanwhile, place the maple syrup, garlic, and soy sauce in a saucepan and heat over medium flame. Wait for it to boil and adjust the heat to low until the sauce thickens.
7. After 15 minutes, take out the Instant Crisp Air Fryer's florets and place them in the saucepan.
8. Toss to coat the florets and place inside the Instant Crisp Air Fryer and cook for another 5 minutes.

Nutrition:

- Calories: 154
- Fat: 2.3g
- Protein: 4.6g

126. Crispy Roasted Broccoli

Difficulty: Easy
Preparation Time: 10 minutes
Cooking Time: 8 minutes
Servings: 1
Ingredients:

- 1/4 Tsp. Masala (½ condiment)
- ½ Tsp. Red chili powder (1 condiment)
- ½ Tsp. Salt (1 condiment)
- 1/4 Tsp. Turmeric powder (½ condiment)
- 1 Tbsp. Chickpea flour (1 healthy fat)
- 1 Tbsp. Yogurt (2 healthy fats)
- ½ Pound broccoli (1green)

Directions:

1. Cut broccoli up into florets. Immerse in a bowl of water with two teaspoons of salt for at least half an hour to remove impurities.
2. Take out broccoli florets from water and let drain. Wipe down thoroughly.
3. Mix all other ingredients to create a marinade.
4. Toss broccoli florets in the marinade. Cover and chill for 15-30 minutes.
5. Preheat the Instant Crisp Air Fryer to 390 degrees. Place marinated broccoli florets into the fryer, lock the air fryer lid, set the temperature to 350°F, and set the time to 10 minutes. Florets will be crispy when done.

Nutrition:

- Calories: 96
- Fat: 1.3g
- Protein: 7g

127. Crispy Cauliflowers

Difficulty: Easy
Preparation Time: 10 Minutes
Cooking Time: 10 Minutes
Servings: 4
Ingredients:

- 2 Cup cauliflower florets, diced (6greens)
- ½ Cup almond flour (1 healthy fat)
- ½ Cup coconut flour (1 healthy fat)
- Salt and pepper to taste (½ condiment)
- 1 Tsp. Mixed herbs (1green)
- 1 Tsp. Chives, chopped (1green)
- 1 Egg (1 lean)
- 1 Tsp. Cumin (1 condiment)
- ½ Tsp. Garlic powder (1 condiment)
- 1 Cup water (1 condiment)
- Oil for frying (1 condiment)

Directions:

1. Combine the egg, salt, garlic, water, cumin, chives, mixed herbs, pepper, and flour in a mixing bowl.
2. Stir in the cauliflower to the mixture and then fry them in oil until they become golden in color.
3. Serve.

Nutrition:

- Protein: 3.3g
- Fat: 10.4g
- Calories: 259

128. Red Pepper & Kale Air Fried Egg Muffins

Difficulty: Average
Preparation Time: 10 Minutes
Cooking Time: 25 Minutes
Servings: 2
Ingredients:
For the Egg Muffin:

- 4 Eggs (1 healthy fat)
- 1 Cup Liquid egg whites (½ healthy fat)
- ¼ Cup Greek yogurt, plain, low fat (1/4 healthy fat)
- ¼ Tsp. Salt (1/4 condiment)

For the Red Bell Pepper, Goat Cheese & Kale Mix:

- 6 oz. Red bell pepper, cored and chopped (3greens)
- 5 oz. Kale, frozen, chopped (2greens)
- 1 oz. Goat cheese (½ healthy fat)

Directions:

1. Thaw the frozen cauliflower rice for 10 minutes.
2. Preheat the air fryer to 190°C.
3. In a large bowl, combine Greek yogurt, egg whites, eggs, cheese, and salt.
4. Add all the vegetables to the bowl mix to combine well.
5. Take 12 muffin tins and lightly spray with cooking oil.
6. Transfer the mixture evenly into the muffin tins.
7. Place them in the air fryer and bake for 25 minutes until the center portion becomes hard.
8. Do a toothpick test by inserting it in the center and check if it comes out clean.
9. Take it out from the air fryer and allow it to settle down the heat before serving.
10. Enjoy your muffin.

Nutrition:

- Calories: 323
- Fat: 15.4g
- Protein: 34g

Chapter 11. Side Dish Recipes

129. Low Carb Air-Fried Calzones

Preparation Time: 15 Minutes
Cooking Time: 27 Minutes
Servings: 2
Ingredients:

- 1/3 Cup cooked chicken breast (shredded)
- One teaspoon olive oil
- 3 Cups Spinach leaves (baby)
- Whole-wheat pizza dough, freshly prepared
- 1/3 Cup Marinara sauce (lower-sodium)
- 1/4 Cup Diced red onion
- 6 Tbsp. Skim mozzarella cheese
- Cooking spray

Directions:

1. In a medium skillet, over a medium flame, add oil, onions. Sauté until soft. Then add spinach leaves, cook until wilted. Turn off the heat and add chicken and marinara sauce.
2. Cut the dough into two pieces.
3. Add 1/4 of the spinach mix on each circle dough piece.
4. Add skim shredded cheese on top. Fold the dough over and crimp the edges.
5. Spray the calzones with cooking spray.
6. Put calzones in the air fryer. Cook for 12 minutes, at 325°F, until the dough is light brown. Turn the calzone over and cook for eight more minutes.

Nutrition:

- Calories: 348
- Fat: 12g
- Protein: 21g
- Carbohydrate: 18g

130. Air-Fried Tortilla Hawaiian Pizza

Preparation Time: 10 Minutes
Cooking Time: 20 Minutes
Servings: 1
Ingredients:

- Mozzarella Cheese
- Tortilla wrap
- 1 Tbsp. Tomato sauce

Toppings:

- 2 Tbsp. Cooked chicken shredded or hotdog
- 3 Tbsp. Pineapple pieces
- Half slice of ham, cut into pieces
- Cheese slice cut into pieces

Directions:

1. Lay a tortilla flat on a plate, add tomato sauce, and spread it.
2. Add some shredded mozzarella, add toppings. Top with cheese slices
3. Put in the air fryer and cook for five or ten minutes at 160 C.
4. Take out from the air fryer and slice it. Serve hot with baby spinach.

Nutrition:

- Calories: 178
- Proteins: 21g
- Carbs: 15g
- Fat: 15g

131. Tasty Kale & Celery Crackers

Preparation Time: 10 Minutes
Cooking Time: 20 Minutes
Servings: 2
Ingredients:

- 1 Cup of flax seeds, ground
- 1 Cup flax seeds, soaked overnight and drained
- 2 Bunches kale, chopped
- 1 Bunch basil, chopped
- ½ Bunch celery, chopped
- 2 Garlic cloves, minced
- 1/3 Cup olive oil

Directions:

1. Mix the ground flaxseed with celery, kale, basil, and garlic in your food processor and mix well.
2. Add the oil and soaked flaxseed, then mix again, scatter in the pan of your air fryer, break into medium crackers and cook for 20 minutes at 380 degrees F.
3. Serve as an appetizer and break into cups.
4. Enjoy

Nutrition:

- Calories: 143
- Fat: 1g
- Fiber: 2g
- Carbs: 8g
- Protein: 4g

132. Air Fryer Personal Mini Pizza

Preparation Time: 2 Minutes
Cooking Time: 5 Minutes
Servings: 1
Ingredients:

- 1/4 Cup Sliced olives
- 1 Pita bread
- 1 Tomato
- ½ Cup Shredded cheese

Directions:

1. Let the air fryer preheat to 350°F
2. Lay the pita flat on a plate. Add cheese, slices of tomatoes, and olives.
3. Cook for five minutes at 350°F
4. Take the pizza out of the air fryer.
5. Slice it and enjoy.

Nutrition:

- Calories: 344kcal
- Carbohydrates: 37g
- Protein: 18g
- Fat: 13g

133. Air Fried Cheesy Chicken Omelet

Preparation Time: 5 Minutes
Cooking Time: 18 Minutes
Servings: 2
Ingredients:

- ½ Cup cooked chicken breast, (diced) divided
- 4 Eggs
- 1/4 Tsp. Onion powder, divided
- ½ Tsp. Salt, divided
- 1/4 Tsp. Pepper divided
- 2 Tbsp. Shredded cheese divided
- 1/4 Tsp. Granulated garlic, divided

Directions:

1. Take two ramekins, grease them with olive oil.
2. Add two eggs to each ramekin. Add cheese with seasoning.
3. Blend to combine. Add 1/4 cup of cooked chicken on top.
4. Cook for 14-18 minutes, in the air fryer at 330°F, or until fully cooked.

Nutrition:

- Calories: 185
- Proteins: 20g
- Carbs: 10g
- Fat: 5g

134. 5-Ingredients Air Fryer Lemon Chicken

Preparation Time: 5 Minutes
Cooking Time: 15 Minutes
Servings: 4
Ingredients:

- 1 and ½ cups Whole-wheat crumbs
- 6 Pieces of chicken tenderloins
- Two eggs
- Two half lemons and lemon slices
- Kosher salt to taste

Directions:

1. In a dish, whisk the eggs.
2. In a separate dish, add the breadcrumbs.
3. With egg, coat the chicken and roll in breadcrumbs.
4. Add the breaded chicken to the air fryer.
5. Cook for 14 minutes at 400°F, flip the chicken halfway through.
6. Take out from air fryer and squeeze lemon juice and sprinkle with kosher salt and Serve with lemon slices.

Nutrition:

- Cal: 240
- Fat: 12g
- Net Carbs: 13g
- Protein: 27g

135. Air Fryer Popcorn Chicken

Preparation Time: 10 Minutes
Cooking Time: 20 Minutes
Servings: 2
Ingredients:
For the marinade:

- 8 Cups chicken tenders, cut into bite-size pieces
- ½ Tsp. Freshly ground black pepper
- 2 Cups Almond milk
- 1 Tsp. Salt
- ½ Tsp. Paprika

Dry Mix:

- 3 Tsp. Salt
- 3 Cups Flour
- 2 Tsp. Paprika
- Oil spray
- 2 Tsp. Freshly ground black pepper

Directions:

1. In a bowl, add all marinade ingredients and chicken. Mix well, and put it in a Ziplock bag, and refrigerate for two hours for the minimum, or six hours.

2. In a large bowl, add all the dry ingredients.
3. Coat the marinated chicken to the dry mix. Into the marinade again, then for the second time in the dry mixture.
4. Spray the air fryer basket with olive oil and place the breaded chicken pieces in one single layer. Spray oil over the chicken pieces too.
5. Cook at 370 degrees for 10 minutes, tossing halfway through.
6. Serve immediately with salad greens or dipping sauce.

Nutrition:

- Calories: 340
- Proteins: 20g
- Carbs: 14g
- Fat: 10g

136. Air Fryer Chicken Nuggets

Preparation Time: 15 Minutes
Cooking Time: 15 Minutes
Servings: 4
Ingredients:

- Olive oil spray
- 2 Chicken breasts, skinless boneless, cut into bite pieces
- ½ Tsp. of kosher salt& freshly ground black pepper, to taste 2
- Tablespoons Grated parmesan cheese
- 6 Tablespoons Italian seasoned breadcrumbs (whole wheat)
- 2 Tablespoons whole wheat breadcrumbs
- 2 Teaspoons olive oil
- Panko, optional

Directions:

1. Let the air fryer preheat for 8 minutes to 400°F

2. In a big mixing bowl, add panko, parmesan cheese, and breadcrumbs and mix well.
3. Sprinkle kosher salt and pepper on chicken and olive oil; mix well.
4. Take a few pieces of chicken, dunk them into the breadcrumbs mixture.
5. Put these pieces in an air fryer and spray with olive oil.
6. Cook for 8 minutes, turning halfway through
7. Enjoy with kale chips.

Nutrition:

- Calories: 188kcal
- Carbohydrates: 8g
- Protein: 25g
- Fat: 4.5g

137. Air Fryer Sweet & Sour Chicken

Preparation Time: 5 Minutes
Cooking Time: 10 Minutes
Servings: 2
Ingredients:
Chicken:

- 4 Cups chicken breasts/thighs, cut into one-inch pieces
- 2 Tablespoons cornstarch

Sweet & Sour Sauce:

- 2 Tablespoons cornstarch
- 1 Cup pineapple juice
- 2 Tablespoons water
- Half honey cup
- 1 Tablespoon soy sauce
- 3 Tablespoons rice wine vinegar
- 1/4 Teaspoon ground ginger

Optional:

- 1/4 Cup pineapple chunks
- 3-4 Drops of red food coloring (for traditional orange look)

Directions:

1. Let the air fryer preheat to 400 degrees.
2. Coat the chicken in cornstarch until the chicken is coated completely.
3. Put the chicken in the air fryer and let it cook for 7, 9 minutes. Take it out from the air fryer
4. In the meantime, in a saucepan, add pineapple juice, ginger, honey, soy sauce, and rice wine vinegar and cook. Let it simmer for five minutes.
5. Make cornstarch slurry and add in the sauce. Let it simmer for one minute.
6. Coat cooked chicken pieces and servings with steamed vegetables

Nutrition:

- Cal: 302
- Fat: 8g
- Carbs: 18
- Protein: 22g

138. Low Carb Chicken Tenders

Preparation Time: 10 Minutes
Cooking Time: 20 Minutes
Servings: 3
Ingredients:

- 4 Cups Chicken tenderloins
- 1 Egg
- ½ Cup Superfine Almond Flour
- ½ Cup Powdered Parmesan cheese
- ½ Teaspoon Kosher Sea salt
- 1-Teaspoon freshly ground black pepper
- ½ Teaspoon Cajun seasoning

Directions:

1. On a small plate, pour the beaten egg.
2. Mix all ingredients in a zip lock bag, cheese, almond flour, freshly ground black pepper, kosher salt, and other seasonings.
3. Spray the air fryer with oil spray.
4. To avoid clumpy fingers with breading and egg, use different hands. Dip each tender in egg and then in bread until they are all breaded.
5. Use a fork to place one tender at a time, bring it in the zip lock bag, and shake the bag forcefully, make sure all the tenders are covered in almond mixture
6. Use the fork to take out the tender and place it in your air fryer basket.
7. Spray oil on the tenders.
8. Cook for 12 minutes at 350°F or before 160°F registers within. Raise the temperature to 40°F to shade the surface for 3 minutes.
9. Serve with sauce.

Nutrition:

- Calories: 280
- Proteins 20g
- Carbs: 6g|
- Fat: 10g
- Fiber: 5g

139. Cheesy Cauliflower Tots

Preparation Time: 15 Minutes
Cooking Time: 12 Minutes
Servings: 4
Ingredients:

- 1 Large cauliflower head
- 1 Cup shredded mozzarella cheese
- ½ Cup grated Parmesan cheese
- 1 Large egg
- 1/4 Teaspoon garlic powder
- 1/4 Teaspoon dried parsley
- 1/8 Teaspoon onion powder

Directions:

1. Fill a big pot with 2 cups of water on the stovetop, and insert a steamer in the oven. Put to boil bath.
2. Break the cauliflower into pieces and place them on the steamer box—cover the pot and lid.
3. Let steam the cauliflower for 7 minutes until the fork-tender point. Put in a cheesecloth or clean kitchen towel on the steamer basket and let it cool.
4. Push on the sink to eliminate as much extra humidity as possible. If all of the moisture is not removed, the mixture will be too soft to form into tots.
5. Mash down to a smooth consistency with a blade.
6. In a large mixing bowl, put the cauliflower and add the mozzarella, parmesan, egg, garlic powder, parsley, and onion powder. Remove until well combined. The blend should be smooth but easy to mold.
7. Take two tablespoons of the mixture and roll the mixture into a tot form. Repeat with the rest of the mixture. Put the basket into the air fryer.
8. Set the temperature to 320°F and adjust the timer for 12 minutes.
9. Turn the tots halfway through the period of cooking.
10. Cauliflower tots should be golden when fully cooked. Serve warm.

Nutrition:

- Calories: 181
- Protein 13.5g
- Fiber: 3.0g
- Carbohydrates: 6.6g
- Fat: 9.5g|

Chapter 18. Dessert Recipes

140. Bread Dough and Amaretto Dessert

Preparation Time: 15 Minutes
Cooking Time: 8 Minutes
Servings: 12
Ingredients:

- 1 lb. Bread dough
- 1 Cup sugar
- ½ Cup butter
- 1 Cup heavy cream
- 12 oz. Chocolate chips
- 2 Tbsp. amaretto liqueur

Directions:

1. Turn dough, cut into 20 slices and cut each piece in halves.
2. Put the dough pieces with spray sugar and butter, put this into the air fryer's basket, and cook them at 350°F for 5 minutes. Turn them, cook for 3 minutes still. Move to a platter.
3. Melt the heavy cream in a pan over medium heat, put chocolate chips and turn until they melt.
4. Put in liqueur, turn and move to a bowl.
5. Serve bread dippers with the sauce.

Nutrition:

- Calories: 179
- Total Fat: 18g
- Total carbs: 17g

141. Bread Pudding

Preparation Time: 10 Minutes
Cooking Time: 10 Minutes
Servings: 4
Ingredients:

- 6 Glazed doughnuts
- 1 Cup cherries
- 4 Egg yolks
- 1 and ½ Cups whipping cream
- ½ Cup raisins
- ¼ Cup sugar
- ½ Cup chocolate chips

Directions:

1. Mix in cherries with whipping cream and egg in a bowl, then turn properly.
2. Mix in raisins with chocolate chips, sugar, and doughnuts in a bowl, then stir.
3. Combine the two mixtures, pour into an oiled pan, then into the air fryer, and cook at 310°F for 1 hour.
4. Cool pudding before cutting.
5. Serve.

Nutrition:

- Calories: 456
- Total Fat: 11g
- Total carbs: 6g

142. Wrapped Pears

Preparation Time: 10 Minutes
Cooking Time: 10 Minutes
Servings: 4
Ingredients:

- 4 Puff pastry sheets
- 14 oz. Vanilla custard
- 2 Pears
- 1 Egg
- ½ Tbsp. cinnamon powder
- 2 Tbsp. sugar

Directions:

1. Put wisp pastry slices on a flat surface, add a spoonful of vanilla custard at the center of each, add pear halves and wrap.
2. Combine pears with egg, cinnamon, and spray sugar, put into the air fryer's basket, then cook at 320°F for 15 minutes.
3. Split portions on plates.
4. Serve.

Nutrition:

- Calories: 285
- Total Fat: 14g
- Total carbs: 30g

143. Air Fried Bananas

Preparation Time: 5 Minutes
Cooking Time: 10 Minutes
Servings: 4
Ingredients:

- 3 Tbsp. butter
- 2 Eggs
- 8 Bananas
- ½ Cup corn flour
- 3 Tbsp. cinnamon sugar
- 1 Cup panko

Directions:

1. Heat a pan with the butter over medium heat, put panko, turn and cook for 4 minutes, then move to a bowl.
2. Dredge each in flour, panko, and egg mixture, place in the basket of the air fryer, gratinate with cinnamon sugar, and cook at 280°F for 10 minutes.
3. Serve immediately.

Nutrition:

- Calories: 337
- Total fat: 3g
- Total carbs: 23g

144. Tasty Banana Cake

Preparation Time: 10 Minutes
Cooking Time: 30 Minutes
Servings: 4
Ingredients:

- 1 Tbsp. butter, soft
- 1 Egg
- 1/3 Cup brown sugar
- 2 Tbsp. honey
- 1 Banana
- 1 Cup white flour
- 1 Tbsp. baking powder
- ½ Tbsp. cinnamon powder
- Cooking spray

Directions:

1. Grease the cake pan with cooking spray.
2. Mix in butter with honey, sugar, banana, cinnamon, egg, flour, and baking powder in a bowl, then beat.
3. Put the mix in a cake pan with cooking spray, put into the air fryer, and cook at 350°F for 30 minutes.
4. Allow to cool, then slice it.
5. Serve.

Nutrition:

- Calories: 435
- Total Fat: 7g
- Total carbs: 15g

145. Peanut Butter Fudge

Preparation Time: 10 Minutes
Cooking Time: 10 Minutes
Servings: 20
Ingredients:

- 1/4 Cup almonds, toasted and chopped
- 12 oz. Smooth peanut butter
- 15 Drops liquid stevia
- 3 Tbsp. coconut oil
- 4 Tbsp. coconut cream
- Pinch of salt

Directions:

1. Line a baking tray with parchment paper.
2. Melt coconut oil in a pan over low heat. Add peanut butter, coconut cream, stevia, and salt to a saucepan. Stir well.
3. Pour fudge mixture into the prepared baking tray and sprinkle chopped almonds on top.
4. Place the tray in the refrigerator for 1 hour or until set.
5. Slice and serve.

Nutrition:

- Calories: 131
- Fat: 12g
- Carbs: 4g
- Sugar: 2g
- Protein: 5g
- Cholesterol: 0mg

146. Cocoa Cake

Preparation Time: 5 Minutes
Cooking Time: 17 Minutes
Servings: 6
Ingredients:

- 4 oz. Butter

- 3 Eggs
- 3 oz. Sugar
- 1 Tbsp. cocoa powder
- 3 oz. Flour
- ½ Tbsp. lemon juice

Directions:

1. Mix in 1 tablespoon butter with cocoa powder in a bowl and beat.
2. Mix in the rest of the butter with eggs, flour, sugar, and lemon juice in another bowl, blend properly and move the half into a cake pan
3. Put half of the cocoa blend, spread, add the rest of the butter layer, and crest with remaining cocoa.
4. Put into the air fryer and cook at 360° F for 17 minutes.
5. Allow it to cool before slicing.
6. Serve.

Nutrition:

- Calories: 221
- Total Fat: 5g
- Total carbs: 12g

147. Avocado Pudding

Preparation Time: 20 Minutes
Cooking Time: 0 Minutes
Servings: 8
Ingredients:

- 2 Ripe avocados, pitted and cut into pieces
- 1 Tbsp. fresh lime juice
- 14 oz. Can coconut milk
- 2 Tsp. liquid stevia
- 2 Tsp. vanilla

Directions:

1. Inside the blender, add all ingredients and blend until smooth.
2. Serve immediately and enjoy.

Nutrition:

- Calories: 317
- Fat: 30g
- Carbs: 9g
- Sugar: 0.5g
- Protein: 3g
- Cholesterol: 0mg

148. Bounty Bars

Preparation Time: 20 Minutes
Cooking Time: 0 Minutes
Servings: 12
Ingredients:

- 1 Cup coconut cream
- 3 Cups shredded unsweetened coconut
- 1/4 Cup extra virgin coconut oil
- ½ Teaspoon vanilla powder
- 1/4 Cup powdered erythritol
- 1 ½ oz. Cocoa butter
- 5 oz. Dark chocolate

Directions:

1. Heat the oven at 350°F and toast the coconut in it for 5-6 minutes. Remove from the oven once toasted and set aside to cool.
2. Take a bowl of medium size and add coconut oil, coconut cream, vanilla, erythritol, and shredded coconut. Mix the ingredients well to prepare a smooth mixture.
3. Make 12 bars of equal size with the help of your hands from the prepared mixture and adjust in the tray lined with parchment paper.
4. Place the tray in the fridge for around one hour and, in the meantime, put the cocoa butter and dark chocolate in a glass bowl.
5. Heat a cup of water in a saucepan over medium heat and place the bowl over it to melt the cocoa butter and the dark chocolate.
6. Remove from the heat once melted properly, mix well until blended, and set it aside to cool.
7. Take the coconut bars and coat them with dark chocolate mixture one by one using a wooden stick. Adjust on the tray lined with parchment paper and drizzle the remaining mixture over them.
8. Refrigerate for around one hour before you serve the delicious bounty bars.

Nutrition:

- Calories: 230
- Fat: 25g
- Carbohydrates: 5g
- Protein: 32g

149. Simple Cheesecake

Preparation Time: 10 Minutes
Cooking Time: 15 Minutes
Servings: 15
Ingredients:

- 1 lb. Cream cheese
- ½ Tbsp. vanilla extract
- 2 Eggs
- 4 Tbsp. sugar
- 1 Cup graham crackers
- 2 Tbsp. butter

Directions:

1. Mix in butter with crackers in a bowl.
2. Compress crackers blend to the bottom of a cake pan, put into the air fryer, and cook at 350°F for 4 minutes.
3. Mix cream cheese with sugar, vanilla, egg in a bowl and beat properly.
4. Sprinkle filling on crackers crust and cook the cheesecake in the air fryer at 310°F for 15 minutes.
5. Keep the cake in the fridge for 3 hours, slice.
6. Serve.

Nutrition:

- Calories: 257
- Total Fat: 18g
- Total carbs: 22g

150. Chocolate Almond Butter Brownie

Preparation Time: 10 Minutes
Cooking Time: 16 Minutes
Servings: 4
Ingredients:

- 1 Cup bananas, overripe
- ½ Cup almond butter, melted
- 1 Scoop protein powder
- 2 Tbsp. unsweetened cocoa powder

Directions:

1. Preheat the air fryer to 325°F. Grease the air fryer baking pan and set it aside.
2. Blend all ingredients in a blender until smooth.
3. Pour the batter into the prepared pan and place it in the air fryer basket to cook for 16 minutes.
4. Serve and enjoy.

Nutrition:

- Calories: 82
- Fat: 2g
- Carbs: 11g
- Sugar: 5g
- Protein: 7g
- Cholesterol: 16mg

151. Almond Butter Fudge

Preparation Time: 10 Minutes
Cooking Time: 10 Minutes
Servings: 18
Ingredients:

- 3/4 Cup creamy almond butter
- 1 ½ Cups unsweetened chocolate chips

Directions:

1. Line 8x4-inch pan with parchment paper and set aside.
2. Add chocolate chips and almond butter into the double boiler and cook over medium heat until the chocolate-butter mixture is melted. Stir well.
3. Place the mixture into the prepared pan and place in the freezer until set.
4. Slice and serve.

Nutrition:

- Calories: 197
- Fat: 16g
- Carbs: 7g
- Sugar: 1g
- Protein: 4g
- Cholesterol: 0mg

152. Apple Bread

Preparation Time: 5 Minutes
Cooking Time: 40 Minutes
Servings: 6
Ingredients:

- 3 Cups apples
- 1 Cup sugar
- 1 Tbsp. vanilla
- 2 Eggs
- 1 Tbsp. apple pie spice
- 2 Cups white flour
- 1 Tbsp. baking powder
- 1 Butter stick
- 1 Cup water

Directions:

1. Mix the eggs with one butter stick, sugar, vanilla, and apple pie spice, then turn using a mixer.
2. Put apples and turn properly.
3. Mix baking powder with flour in another bowl and turn.
4. Blend the two mixtures, turn and move it to a springform pan.
5. Put the pan into the air fryer and cook at 320°F for 40 minutes
6. Slice.
7. Serve.

Nutrition:

- Calories: 401
- Total Fat: 9g
- Total carbs: 29g

153. Banana Bread

Preparation Time: 5 Minutes
Cooking Time: 40 Minutes
Servings: 6
Ingredients:

- ¾ Cup sugar
- 1/3 Cup butter
- 1 Tbsp. vanilla extract
- 1 Egg
- 2 Bananas
- 1 Tbsp. baking powder
- 1 and ½ Cups flour
- ½ Tbsp. baking soda
- 1/3 Cup milk
- 1 and ½ Tbsp. cream of tartar
- Cooking spray

Directions:

1. Mix the milk with cream of tartar, vanilla, egg, sugar, bananas, and butter in a bowl, then mix all.
2. Mix in flour with baking soda and baking powder.
3. Blend the two mixtures, turn properly, move into an oiled pan with cooking spray, put into the air fryer, and cook at 320°F for 40 minutes.
4. Remove the bread, allow to cool, slice.
5. Serve.

Nutrition:

- Calories: 540
- Total Fat: 16g
- Total carbs: 28g

154. Mini Lava Cakes

Preparation Time: 5 Minutes
Cooking Time: 20 Minutes
Servings: 3
Ingredients:

- 1 Egg
- 4 Tbsp. sugar
- 2 Tbsp. olive oil
- 4 Tbsp. milk
- 4 Tbsp. flour
- 1 Tbsp. cocoa powder
- ½ Tbsp. baking powder
- ½ Tbsp. orange zest
- A pinch of salt

Directions:

1. Mix in egg with sugar, flour, salt, oil, milk, orange zest, baking powder, and cocoa powder, turn properly. Move it to oiled ramekins.
2. Put ramekins in the air fryer and cook at 320°F for 20 minutes.
3. Serve warm.

Nutrition:

- Calories: 329
- Total Fat: 8.5g
- Total carbs: 12.4g

155. Ricotta Ramekins

Preparation Time: 10 Minutes
Cooking Time: 1 Hour
Servings: 4
Ingredients:

- 6 Eggs, whisked
- 1 and ½ Pounds ricotta cheese, soft
- ½ Pound stevia
- 1 Teaspoon vanilla extract
- ½ Teaspoon baking powder
- Cooking spray

Directions:

1. In a bowl, mix the eggs with the ricotta and the other ingredients except for the cooking spray and whisk well.
2. Grease 4 ramekins with the cooking spray, pour the ricotta cream in each and bake at 360 degrees F for 1 hour.
3. Serve cold.

Nutrition:

- Calories: 180
- Fat: 5.3
- Fiber: 5.4
- Carbs: 11.5
- Protein: 4

156. Strawberry Sorbet

Preparation Time: 15 Minutes
Cooking Time: 10 Minutes
Servings: 6
Ingredients:

- 1 Cup strawberries, chopped
- 1 Tablespoon of liquid honey
- 2 Tablespoons water
- 1 Tablespoon lemon juice

Directions:

1. Preheat the water and liquid honey until you get a homogenous liquid.
2. Blend the strawberries until smooth and combine them with the honey liquid and lemon juice.
3. Transfer the strawberry mixture to the ice cream maker and churn it for 20 minutes or until the sorbet is thick.
4. Scoop the cooked sorbet in the ice cream cups.

Nutrition:

- Calories: 30
- Fat: 0.4g
- Fiber: 1.4g
- Carbs: 14.9g
- Protein: 0.9g

157. Crispy Apples

Preparation Time: 10 Minutes
Cooking Time: 10 Minutes
Servings: 4
Ingredients:

- 2 Tbsp. cinnamon powder
- 5 Apples
- ½ Tbsp. nutmeg powder
- 1 Tbsp. maple syrup
- ½ Cup water
- 4 Tbsp. butter
- ¼ Cup flour
- ¾ Cup oats
- ¼ Cup brown sugar

Directions:

1. Get the apples in a pan, put in nutmeg, maple syrup, cinnamon, and water.
2. Mix in butter with flour, sugar, salt, and oat, turn, put a spoonful of the blend over apples, get into the air fryer and cook at 350°F for 10 minutes.
3. Serve while warm.

Nutrition:

- Calories: 387
- Total Fat: 5.6g
- Total carbs: 12.4g

158. Cocoa Cookies

Preparation Time: 10 Minutes
Cooking Time: 14 Minutes
Servings: 12
Ingredients:

- 6 oz. Coconut oil
- 6 Eggs
- 3 oz. Cocoa powder
- 2 Tbsp. vanilla
- ½ Tbsp. baking powder
- 4 oz. Cream cheese
- 5 Tbsp. sugar

Directions:

1. Mix the eggs with sugar, coconut oil, baking powder, cocoa powder, cream cheese, vanilla in a blender, then sway and turn using a mixer.
2. Get it into a lined baking dish and put it into the fryer at 320°F, and bake for 14 minutes.
3. Split cookie sheet into rectangles.
4. Serve.

Nutrition:

- Calories: 149
- Total Fat: 2.4g
- Total carbs: 27.2g

159. Cinnamon Pears

Preparation Time: 2 Hours
Cooking Time: 0 Minutes
Servings: 6
Ingredients:

- 2 Pears
- 1 Teaspoon ground cinnamon
- 1 Tablespoon Erythritol
- 1 Teaspoon liquid stevia
- 4 Teaspoons butter

Directions:

1. Cut the pears on the halves.
2. Then scoop the seeds from the pears with the help of the scooper.
3. In a shallow bowl, mix up together Erythritol and ground cinnamon.
4. Sprinkle every pear half with cinnamon mixture and drizzle with liquid stevia.
5. Then add butter and wrap in the foil.
6. Bake the pears for 25 minutes at 365°F.
7. Then remove the pears from the foil and transfer them to the serving plates.

Nutrition:

- Calories: 96
- Fat: 4.4g
- Fiber: 1.4g
- Carbs: 3.9g
- Protein: 0.9g

160. Cherry Compote

Preparation Time: 2 Hours
Cooking Time: 0 Minutes
Servings: 6
Ingredients:

- 2 Peaches, pitted, halved
- 1 Cup cherries, pitted
- ½ Cup grape juice
- ½ Cup strawberries
- 1 Tablespoon liquid honey
- 1 Teaspoon vanilla extract
- 1 Teaspoon ground cinnamon

Directions:

1. Pour grape juice into the saucepan.
2. Add vanilla extract and ground cinnamon. Bring the liquid to a boil.
3. After this, put peaches, cherries, and strawberries in the hot grape juice and bring them to a boil.
4. Remove the mixture from heat, add liquid honey, and close the lid.
5. Let the compote rest for 20 minutes.
6. Carefully mix up the compote and transfer it to the serving plate.

Nutrition:

- Calories: 80
- Fat: 0.4g
- Fiber: 2.4g
- Carbs: 19.9g
- Protein: 0.9g

CPSIA information can be obtained
at www.ICGtesting.com
Printed in the USA
BVHW040909100621
609274BV00013B/2868

9 781802 430844